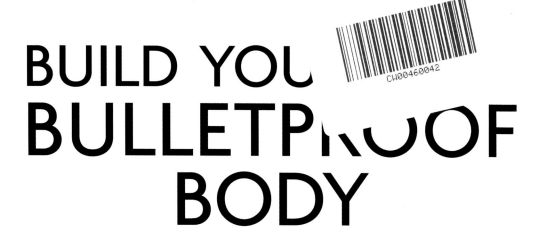

BUILD YOU BULLETPROOF BODY

BODY

Bodyweight Exercises for
Strength, Resilience and Injury Prevention

Revised Edition

ROSS CLIFFORD & ASHLEY KALYM

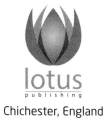

lotus
publishing

Chichester, England

First published in 2018. Revised edition published in 2022 by
Lotus Publishing
Apple Tree Cottage, Inlands Road, Nutbourne, Chichester, PO18 8RJ

Anatomical Drawings Amanda Williams
Photographs Fiona Hook
Text Design Medlar Publishing Solutions Pvt Ltd., India
Cover Design Jim Wilkie
Printed and Bound in the UK by Short Run Press Limited

British Library Cataloguing-in-Publication Data
A CIP record for this book is available from the British Library
ISBN 978 1 913088 30 9

Contents

Abbreviations

ACL	Anterior cruciate ligament
ITB	Iliotibial band
LCL	Lateral collateral ligament
MCL	Medial collateral ligament
PCL	Posterior cruciate ligament
PFPS	Patellofemoral pain syndrome
ROM	Range of motion

Preface

There has never been a better time to be involved in body-weight exercise. Over the last few years, body-weight training has held a top five position in the list of top fitness trends. But unlike wearable technology, which currently sits in first place, body-weight training is not really a trend. It is not new, and it is definitely not a fad that will fade into obscurity in the years to come. Although bodyweight exercise has been around for thousands of years as a formal training method, it existed long before this when humans increased their survival chances with running, climbing, jumping and lifting activities. It almost seems instinctive to us to use the weight of our bodies as a form of resistance.

In today's world, body-weight training is no longer an exercise option but instead a thriving community of people who value their physical function over a purely aesthetic outcome. Myriad online facilities now exist to take you from the most fundamental of human body movements through to spectacular feats of strength and flexibility, such as the human flag. There are groups that exist, bestowing kudos on their global members who achieve the Holy Grail that is the muscle-up. High-quality calisthenics books are available to explain and illustrate a range of progressive techniques and routines to suit both the novice and the expert fitness fan.

The focus of body-weight exercise has long been the development of strength, but many of the exercises will also develop mobility around joints and flexibility of muscles. This is largely because the exercises do not isolate muscle groups and immobilise large parts of the body; instead, body-weight training uses most of the body at any time while focusing the load on specific body areas. Often this requires the support of the core or stabilising muscles. All of this can be done anywhere and with a minimal amount of equipment, making it accessible in terms of location, cost and time. What more could you want?

The nature of this book differs slightly from the focus of most other body-weight training manuals and online facilities. It is the result of a partnership between a chartered physiotherapist and a calisthenics expert who have long appreciated the use of body-weight exercise in developing physical resilience to the strains of modern living, and the potential for these exercises to rehabilitate injuries that have already occurred. Without a doubt, if you were to regularly complete the exercises herein, you would develop increased strength, which is the capacity to *generate* force or pressure. But strength can also mean the ability to *withstand* force or pressure. This is the focus of *Bulletproof Bodies* – we combine strength gains with the concept of physical resilience, which is the capacity to recover quickly from physical stress and to spring back from physical difficulty.

Our aim is to demonstrate and *educate* how the principles of body-weight exercise can be applied to the prevention and rehabilitation of injuries in the musculoskeletal system. No matter how hard you train and how clean you live, you must understand that some injuries are inevitable. We cannot control all events and all external forces, but we can ensure that we are physically robust enough to absorb as much of this force as possible before we reach breaking point. Once broken, however, we must then guide our bodies back to the best function possible. This book will help you in achieving both of these aims.

We hope that this book will give you a deeper understanding and appreciation of the incredible human musculoskeletal system, and that you will come to know your own body better. This is not an academic textbook for trainee health or sports professionals, but is intended as a 'need-to-know' guide to common structures in the body and the problems that can develop. Once we have established this in an accessible way, we offer you a wide range of targeted body-weight exercises to rehabilitate and make resistant specific body areas. At the end of the book, we combine these exercises in set routines as suggestions for developing whole-body physical resilience. All of these exercises are tried and tested by both authors and have been used by us for many years to develop strength and recover from injury.

One final word regarding the exercises: at first sight you may wonder if we have misunderstood the effects of the proposed exercises. The answer is 'no': we have 're-understood' the exercises. For example, you may be familiar with the pull-up as a classic means of increasing size and strength of the back muscles, especially the latissimus dorsi muscles. Take a minute to think through this well-known exercise – gripping the bar, the initial pull at the elbows, and the bend in the elbows required to bring yourself to the bar. You may now be thinking about the forearm 'pump' that you get with this exercise. Now ask yourself – is this just a back-muscle exercise? The answer again is 'no'. Like all body-weight exercise, it is not 'just' anything. We will hopefully help you to see the wider benefits of body-weight exercise and reinterpret the gains available to you with this most fashionable of exercise trends!

Train smart.
**Ross Clifford & Ashley Kalym,
February 2022**

1

Musculoskeletal Injury

Musculoskeletal injuries or disorders can affect muscles, joints, tendons and ligaments in all parts of the body. These issues can happen at any time during the lifetime, in the active and inactive, and can seemingly occur for no known reason. There may be an obvious trauma or injury that is responsible for the disorder, but more likely than not the pain or dysfunction comes on without trauma. It may be sudden, in that you awoke with it, or it may be a slowly worsening niggle that will not go away.

If you currently have such a problem, you are not alone. Musculoskeletal injuries are widespread, with lower back pain being the most common condition, affecting nearly everyone at some point in his or her life. Estimates suggest that in developed countries 4–33% of the population at any given time will experience lower back pain. In some countries, musculoskeletal disorders make up around 40% of work-related illness, suggesting that you are more likely to develop a musculoskeletal problem through your daily routine rather than through any kind of sports injury. It is therefore very likely that at some point in your life, probably in the

not-too-distant future, this book may be of great use to you.

In this first chapter we will briefly look at the soft-tissue repair process, differentiate chronic from acute musculoskeletal problems, and outline general types of chronic musculoskeletal disorders.

▓ Soft-tissue Injury and Repair

If at any point a force is applied to the musculoskeletal structures that exceeds their ability to withstand that force, there will be disruption to the normal structure and function of that tissue. This may be minor and give you nothing more than a dull ache for a day or two. If you are no stranger to exercise or physical work, you may recognise this as muscle soreness, where there has been minor damage to the muscle tissue. With adequate rest and nutrition (see Chapter 4), this ache will subside as the inflammatory process passes and the muscle fibres are repaired and perhaps even made thicker and stronger. All of this is a normal process and happens on a daily basis as our musculoskeletal systems respond to the dynamic ebb and flow of forces applied to our bodies.

This book will focus on musculoskeletal problems more troublesome than muscle soreness, and more specifically on problems that have arisen when internal or external forces applied to body tissues have exceeded their tolerance and led to injury. We will take a broad look at the process of repair that many musculoskeletal structures undergo when injured, and discuss the reasons why some injuries do not fully resolve in the expected timescales. These are referred to as *chronic injuries*, and this book will offer targeted body-weight exercises to rehabilitate and build resilience to these types of injury.

> **KEY POINT** *Soft tissue and bone breakdown and repair happens on a daily basis; it is a normal process that takes place in response to the forces acting on your body.*

Injury and Inflammation

The 'injury' may take many forms, from the obvious stretching trauma of an ankle sprain to the prolonged excessive loading of spinal ligaments and discs. Ultimately, a force has been applied that exceeds the strength of the musculoskeletal structure, causing it to deform or break. Damage may occur to cells, muscle fibres, connective tissue fibres, bone tissue or blood vessels passing through the area. If the trauma is extreme, several of these structures may be disrupted. If blood vessels are damaged, you will develop swelling, which may appear as bruising. Damage to cells and fibres will trigger the inflammatory process; this can also result in swelling, but is usually more delayed and can take several hours or days to develop.

Inflammatory chemicals irritate your nerve endings to cause pain, reminding you that you have an injured body part that needs rest. These chemicals can open blood vessels and make them leaky, leaving the injured area swollen, red and warm. The common advice in these circumstances is **PRICE** – **P**rotect the injured area, **R**est from further aggravating movements, apply **I**ce, **C**ompress the area to limit inflammatory fluid, and **E**levate where possible to allow gravity to aid in the drainage of the swelling. A fuller explanation of this

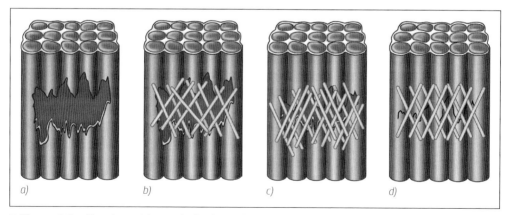

■ **Figure 1.1.** Scar tissue: (a) a tear in the tissue; (b) scar tissue laid down in a random fashion; (c) built-up tension around the area of repair, caused by too much time with lack of movement; (d) scar tissue better aligned to the natural tension in the tissue.

method is not the focus of this book, and so we recommend in such cases that you see a qualified health or medical professional for further advice.

> **KEY POINT** *Inflammatory chemicals irritate your nerve endings to cause pain, reminding you that you have an injured body part that may need a period of relative rest.*

The Repair Process

Inflammation following injury can last from a few hours to several weeks, depending on the severity of the injury. The inflammatory process is essential in order to 'kick-start' the repair process that begins alongside the inflammatory phase. During this repair process, new material is laid down to replace or bridge the original damaged tissue. In bone, joint lining and skeletal muscle, the new tissue is the same as that lost: it is like-for-like. In connective tissue, however, such as tendons, ligaments and the fibres around muscles, the original tissue is replaced: the 'makeshift' material is commonly known as *scar tissue*. Scar tissue is made of collagen fibres, and this material is the structural foundation of much of the body. Eventually the scar tissue may come to resemble the tissue around it, but it will never be the same. This may lead to ongoing injuries such as a niggling hamstring strain or an ankle ligament sprain.

After a while, the newly laid collagen begins to mature; this may start at around three weeks after injury and last for many months. Links develop between the collagen fibres to strengthen the healing tissue, and the fibres begin to shrink. These last two stages indicate why sometimes the healing process is never fully resolved.

> **KEY POINT** *When connective tissue, such as tendons, ligaments and the fibres around muscles, is damaged, the original tissue is replaced by scar tissue made of collagen.*

When Repair Fails

As the collagen fibres in the healing breach begin to shrink and form strong bonds between themselves, you may be left with an area of scar tissue that is not fit for purpose within an otherwise healthy muscle, ligament or tendon. The fibres of these surrounding tissues will be lined up along the direction of stress, meaning that they can glide and extend under stretch and be able to take up the 'pull'. When scar tissue is laid down, it is done so in a haphazard way, running in all directions. If the healing wound does not undergo gradual loading and movement, the fibres are not 'remodelled' to align with surrounding fibres. The result is that you return to normal movement after a period of rest only to 'pull' the area again, creating more inflammation and more scar tissue. As the healing fibres shrink and strengthen, this also makes the area of injury less able to respond to stress and strain, leading to re-injury, inflammation and scar tissue formation. This cycle can become an ongoing process, as an excess amount of poorly constructed scar tissue is unable to replicate the original tissue. Such a cycle can form the basis of a chronic, ongoing or recurrent musculoskeletal disorder.

■ Differentiating Musculoskeletal Injury

When referring to an illness or injury, the term *chronic* by definition means to persist for long periods or to constantly recur.

This is the basis of our discussion above when looking at scar tissue repair and the dangers of inadequate rehabilitation. Chronic injuries may also be referred to as *overuse injuries*, to distinguish them from injuries that come on quickly after obvious trauma, known as *acute injuries.*

Chronic overuse injuries are seen and experienced more often than acute traumatic injuries, and can easily arise from occupational, sporting or leisure activities. They tend not to be instantly disabling, and their onset is more gradual, with varying degrees of pain and dysfunction. The problem area may worsen with repeated exposure to the aggravating activity; this could be a gym or sporting movement, or more likely the result of sitting for long periods or repeating a manual task for work or leisure.

Chronic overuse injuries often result from a prolonged stress that exceeds the ability of the tissue to withstand that stress. This issue can occur in deconditioned and conditioned bodies, and can depend on the amount of stress, its duration and the nature of its application. Ultimately, we can look at three potential causes:

1. The tissue/body is poorly conditioned in relation to the demands of the task. In this book we focus on developing physical resilience in multiple body areas through functional exercises.
2. The environment has contributed to the injury. Look at the environment, such as desk set-up, driving position or any gym/sporting equipment, to see where changes can be made to ease stress to the body.
3. The activity creates excessive stress. When otherwise fit and healthy people develop lower back pain from sitting, they often want to know what is wrong with their spines. The answer is usually 'nothing'. The human spine is not built for sitting long hours in a position of spinal flexion (bending). Modify the activity.

■ Types of Chronic Musculoskeletal Injury

In Chapters 5 to 11 of this book we cover specific body areas and outline some commonly seen musculoskeletal problems affecting these regions. Many of the disorders discussed are chronic/overuse injuries or were once acute injuries but have failed to reach full repair. Such musculoskeletal disorders can affect muscles, joints, tendons and ligaments in all parts of the body. We will briefly outline here the types of problems that will be explored further in later chapters.

Muscle Strains
Muscle strains can occur throughout the body, but are most common in long muscles that cross two joints; this is because there are multiple demands on the muscle to move or control more than one joint at any one time. Such injuries are often seen in the hamstrings and the calf muscle, both of which are heavily loaded muscles and play an essential role in slowing movement and absorbing force. In the relevant chapters we provide specific exercises to target the function of these muscles in order to create resilience to everyday loads. Strains to both the hamstrings and the calf can become chronic when the scar tissue is not properly rehabilitated. Again, recommended targeted exercises to complete the rehabilitation process will be given.

Tendon Problems
Tendon problems were once considered to be an inflammatory problem, but as you explore the body chapters in this book,

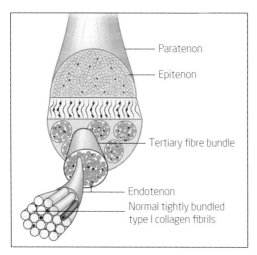

Labels: Paratenon, Epitenon, Tertiary fibre bundle, Endotenon, Normal tightly bundled type I collagen fibrils

■ **Figure 1.2.** Anatomy of a tendon.

you will see that we attribute them more to degeneration of the tendons. This notion is based on current thinking and research in this area, and we offer targeted exercises to help rehabilitate 'tendinopathies' or to develop resilience to developing tendon disorders. Common problematic tendons include those at the shoulder (Chapter 5), the elbow (Chapter 6), the knee (Chapter 9) and the ankle (Chapter 10).

Ligament Problems

Ligament sprains can become chronic if not fully rehabilitated. The scar tissue within the healing ligament may be of poor quality if you have not developed a gradual load through the ligament. When stress is suddenly applied, even with normal activities, you may find that the area swells and becomes painful. Such a problem is commonly seen in the ankle after an 'inversion' sprain. There may even be some instability in the area following ligament injury, and so it is essential that the muscles can react adequately and provide additional support to the joint. We offer targeted exercises to develop resilience and rehabilitation for ligament stability injuries to the shoulder (Chapter 5), the knee (Chapter 9) and the ankle (Chapter 10).

Joint-specific Problems

Finally, it is worth considering joint-related problems. Especially, but not exclusively, in weight-bearing joints, osteoarthritis can develop; this is a relatively common disease in older joints but it is not just an affliction of the elderly. Age may be one factor in joint osteoarthritis, but there are many other contributing factors, such as genetics, obesity and prior injury. Nutrition and hydration may also play a part (Chapter 4). Many people hold the notion that osteoarthritis is a condition that will just get worse, or that movement will aggravate it. Neither of these ideas is necessarily true, and we offer targeted exercise as an evidence-supported form of managing pain and dysfunction from osteoarthritis.

All of the disorders discussed in this chapter can be managed in part with movement and exercise, which is the basis of this book. In the next chapter we will explain why body-weight exercise is a suitable means of developing resilience to injury, as well as a basis for rehabilitating chronic injuries. We hope that you will achieve as much freedom from pain and dysfunction as we have by applying these principles to your lives.

2

Advantages of Body-weight Exercise

At this point it is perhaps worth examining why body-weight exercise is so good for injury prevention and rehabilitation, and why traditional methods are not as effective as they could be. A key reason for the latter is that traditional methods of injury prevention and rehabilitation rely on isolating the targeted body part. Ideally, in order to protect against injury, the body area in question should develop strength through a functional range of motion (ROM). The movements should also focus on supporting and stabilising muscles, and not just on the 'big-gun' movement muscles.

▨ Fundamental Movement

Traditional physical therapies rely on isolated movements, corrective exercise and other practices that do not always maximise rehabilitation by developing multiple body areas in a functional way. The goal of rehabilitation should be simple: to make the body as strong, mobile and injury free as possible. If this goal is achieved, the potential for injury will be reduced, and the rehabilitation of an existing injury will be much quicker.

Take the example of someone who has an injury that prevents them from squatting properly or performing lower body movements. The traditional route would be to introduce some stretching to aid flexibility, build strength using some exercise machines, and perhaps incorporate some movements to encourage the correct firing of the muscles in question. These approaches are all fine in theory but do not address the root problem and client aim of being able to squat.

Consider an approach that involves a variety of methods to achieve the aim, but with the fundamental movement at the heart of the program. In the example above, this would involve squatting-based movements as early as possible, with different progressions built in. Developing the squat through a squatting-based activity would take care of the strength, mobility, flexibility and muscle firing patterns together in a single coordinated method.

Minimal Equipment

Physical therapies, personal training and gym environments can sometimes focus on expensive or complex equipment for the prevention and rehabilitation of injury. This may require ongoing access to such equipment or specialist knowledge in order to achieve your rehabilitation or training goals. In this book we present an alternative option, where most of the movements can be performed either without any equipment, or with equipment that is relatively cheap and readily available. This means that the exercises and methods outlined in this book can be performed in most places, from the home to a hotel room, and are not limited to times of access to specialist apparatus or knowledge. You will see, however, that throughout this book we do advise you seek specialist health or medical attention whenever you are not able to easily identify the cause of your pain or dysfunction. We acknowledge that in these instances there is no substitute for an expert face-to-face opinion.

Natural Movement

Another advantage of using body-weight exercise for the prevention and rehabilitation of injury is that the movements used are based on naturally occurring movements. Moving the joints of the elbow, knee, hip and shoulder through a large range while under load is common in children, but in many cases the ability is lost as we get older. Replicating this movement during exercise in adult life is a logical way to restore functional movement at the joints. Squatting, lunging, pushing, pulling, twisting and stretching are all naturally occurring movements that are used to advantage in body-weight exercise.

In many weighted exercises the goal is to move external weights in ever more elaborate ways, none of which truly replicate the natural human movements that all of us engaged in regularly as children.

Variation

Body-weight exercises can be good for maintaining motivation and interest in exercise in general, owing to the large number of possible exercises that are available. Movements can be joint specific, such as a wrist support, or involve lots of large muscle groups, such as the jump squat. The important thing is that it is very difficult to become bored when you have such a vast number of possible movements to perform in each workout. There are also many different ways of performing body-weight movements, including singly, in circuits, for a period of time, for a number of repetitions, in a progression towards a specific movement, and so on. This means that, even if the same exercises are used, there are many ways to perform those particular exercises. For example, if we take an exercise like the pull-up, there are easily 20 or more different variations that can be performed. Of course, not all of these will be suitable for injury prevention, and some may be beyond your current ability, but the important fact is that a wide range of possibilities and variety is available.

Progression and Regression

Another great feature of body-weight exercise is that the movements can be made more difficult or less difficult without the need for adding new equipment. Making an exercise easier is known as *regression*, and is a very useful concept when injured or after a period of detraining. It can also be useful for those who have never exercised but are keen to make a start. If we take the push-up as an example, this can be made easier in many ways, for example by altering the angle of the body, by dropping to the knees instead of balancing on the toes, and even by reducing the ROM. Conversely, increasing the difficulty of an exercise is known as *progression*. If again we take the push-up as our example, we could increase the ROM, slow down the movement or place the feet on a raised platform, all of which will make the movement more difficult.

3

Getting Started

Before starting any exercise routine, whether preventative, rehabilitative, for gains in strength or for aesthetic purposes, it is always recommended to seek the advice of a suitably qualified health or medical professional. You may be carrying an injury that you are unable to associate with those described in this book, or it may be in an 'acute' stage that requires some initial management before beginning a body-weight exercise program. While the majority of exercises in this book are safe and appropriate, even for the out-of-condition individual, some can be riskier than others if not performed correctly or in the presence of an undiagnosed injury. Visiting a health professional can ensure that you are starting on the right path to rehabilitation. This book will then help to supplement and progress your physical resilience with functional multi-muscle and multi-joint exercises.

■ Basic Physical Requirements

Our endeavour in writing this book was to make it usable by a large proportion of the population, including those who are injured or who are returning to exercise and seeking to protect themselves from injury. Accordingly, there are no real physical requirements or base level of fitness required to start on this journey. For some exercises, a certain level of strength and ability will be beneficial, but this level will reveal itself when you move through the exercises within the book. Guidance is provided throughout on how to modify exercises to suit a range of ability levels. We propose the following grading system for each exercise as it is presented, and we recommend that you attempt exercises that are pitched at your level, or below, as follows:

Level 1: Suitable for any ability level, including those either new to exercise or returning after a long break.

Level 2: Suitable for those with a good base level of fitness and physical function, or above.

Level 3: Suitable for those who train regularly and have a high level of fitness and physical function.

When starting any exercise program, many people are concerned that they may not have adequate physical ability to perform it. To address this apprehension, we have included a wide range of exercises and movements that can be performed by almost anyone, anywhere and with minimal equipment. We present a range of exercises, often with variations, to target a range of abilities. It is impossible for us to take into account the ability of every individual reader, and so it will be up to you to explore and test your physical limits. We recommend starting with the easiest exercises and moving on to the more difficult ones once you have mastered the basics. This way, you will determine your baseline and develop a strong foundation to build upon naturally. Throughout this book, we will remind you that you should not overlook the 'easy' or 'basic' exercises; if you do, it will be at the expense of realising later that there are weaknesses in your base strength and resilience to injury.

The physical requirements for the exercises in this book differ from chapter to chapter. *Strength* refers to the ability of muscles to exert force. The stronger your muscles, the more force you can apply, and the more successful you will be with movements that require strength, such as the pull-up. *Mobility* is simply the ability of your body to move into certain positions without being hindered. For example, the deep squat position is a real test of mobility in the lower body, since most people have the strength but not the mobility to fully assume the position. *Flexibility* refers to the ability of the muscles to allow the joints to move into extreme positions. Touching one's toes is an example of flexibility. As we outlined in the introduction to this book, *resilience* can be thought of as the ability to withstand or respond to the forces applied to the body. We therefore focus on how you can develop strength and mobility to improve your physical resilience.

▉ Making Enough Time

The amount of time you can devote to a regime of injury prevention and rehabilitation will depend on your own personal circumstances in terms of not only how much physical time you have available but also the nature of your injury or injuries. You must also consider the timescale required for you to regain function, whether this be an occupational or sporting demand, or a goal to reduce pain.

We all have 24 hours every day at our disposal; however, with regard to exercise and physical training, the challenge is finding the time within your hectic day to complete your training program. There is no magic answer to this universal problem, but we do offer one piece of advice – work out your priorities. For example, many of us watch some television every day, and this is time that can also be used to exercise. Ask yourself whether you would rather continue with lower back pain or that niggling hamstring, or be up to date with the latest TV drama. The option of training and protecting against injury must always be weighed against the time and effort costs of training. If rehabilitating your sore shoulder is more important to you than watching the latest episode of your favourite television program, then you will likely find time to do it. The fact that many of these exercises can be done daily in your living room for 10 minutes means that you can probably have the best of both worlds!

How much time to devote to injury prevention and rehabilitation will depend on personal circumstances. A niggling ankle injury may only require a few minutes of attention each day, whereas a long-standing lower back problem caused by years of physical neglect or overuse will take more time to rehabilitate and recover.

We recommend that you proceed slowly and build your training from the ground up. If you are already quite active and have a regular physical routine, it will be easy for you to add some of our suggested exercises to your program to protect against or rehabilitate injury. Time spent doing this will not be wasted.

■ Equipment

An effective and solid injury prevention and rehabilitation routine does not require huge amounts of expensive equipment. Nearly all of the exercises we present in this book can be performed without the use of equipment, which makes them accessible and practical for most people. Occasionally there are some exercises that require additional equipment; however, we have kept these to a minimum and ensured that such equipment is either commonly found in most gyms or inexpensive and readily available. The following sections outline the equipment that you might need to perform some of the movements in this book.

Pull-up Bar

A pull-up bar is an essential piece of body-weight exercise apparatus that allows you to manipulate the effect of gravity as the resistance. Exercises benefitting from this piece of equipment include the scapula pull-up,

triceps dip and false-grip hang, to name a few. Pull-up bars can be found in almost any good gym, and they can also be purchased for home use. The criteria that you should look for in this apparatus are: 1) a bar thickness that is comfortable to hold (too thick and it will be difficult to hold onto; too thin and the hands will pinch); 2) a suitable height from the ground, enabling easy and safe access; and 3) a sturdy point of attachment, ensuring your safety.

If you do not have a pull-up bar in your gym, or if you train from home, there are other options available. Pull-up bars for home use are now quite popular, with choices for many different situations. One option is to use a pull-up bar that secures to the doorframe, requiring no screws or bolts of any kind. If this is too temporary, it is possible to fix a pull-up bar to a wall or ceiling (but these obviously require a location that allows this, such as a basement or garage). Another option is a stand-alone unit that has a base and frame that support the bar; these types often come with dip bars as part of the structure, and so they can be a good investment (and are often cheaper than even a six-month gym membership). Alternatively, look for suitable fixed objects that can be found in many parks, which would also allow you to train outdoors.

Foam Roller

Foam rollers are essential for the process known as *foam rolling*, or the technique

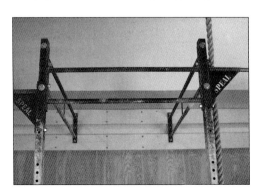

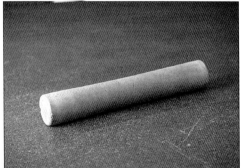

known as *myofascial release*. They come in many different types, ranging from very soft, suited to beginners, to much harder, suitable for those who are more experienced. Foam rollers are also available with a variety of features: some have raised bumps and patterns on them, which are designed to apply a little more pressure than if the roller was smooth. Most gyms these days will have foam rollers, of various types. If the gym you frequent does not have them, or if you train from home, they can be purchased at low cost, either on the Internet or in good sports shops.

Exercise Mat

An exercise mat is recommended, especially for some of the exercises that put pressure on the hands and wrists. They are also useful for performing many of the movements that require you to place your knees on the ground. There are many different types of exercise mat: some are thin and more of a yoga-type mat, while others are thick and more suited to exercise classes. Nearly every gym will have these; if not, they can be found at low cost on the Internet or in good sports shops.

Abdominal Wheel

The abdominal wheel is used for only one exercise in this book, namely the kneeling roll-out. This movement is one of the most demanding core exercises that exists, and can

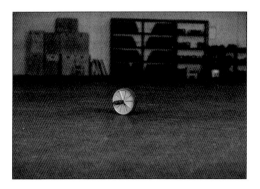

contribute significantly to spinal strength and resilience. The kneeling roll-out is a more advanced exercise, and so you may want to try this when you have mastered many of the other exercises suggested. Abdominal wheels normally consist of a bar with a wheel in the centre. The wheel size will differ depending on the model that is available to you, and the bar will have space for both hands to grip. In our experience, abdominal wheels are not found in every gym, but many do have them. If you find that your local gym does not have abdominal wheels, they can be purchased at low cost on the Internet or in good sports shops. They have no serviceable parts, are very simple and sturdy in construction, and will remain usable for many years.

Dip Bars

Dip bars are used for exercises such as the scapula dip. They can be found in most modern gyms, and have a main feature of parallel bars approximately two feet apart, at about shoulder height from the ground. In gyms they can normally be found as part of a larger frame, usually paired with a pull-up bar.

If you are not a member of a gym, or if you wish to train from home, dip bars can be purchased relatively cheaply. They are different from pull-up bars in that they will need to be fixed to a wall somehow, and will need to be sturdy enough to support your weight safely. Another alternative is to use the backs of two chairs, or other solid objects that will be strong enough and stable enough to support your weight. If you have the space and the funds, the larger pull-up bar frames usually have dip bars attached as well, killing two birds with one stone. Alternatively, check out your local park for suitable equipment.

Exercise Ball

Exercise or gym balls, sometimes called *Swiss balls*, are very common in most gyms (and homes!) around the world. They have become more popular in recent years because of the surge of core training and exercising on unstable surfaces. The gym ball is suggested in this book for a knee exercise, but it can also be used for many other movements that are not discussed in this book. The balls can be purchased at low cost in sports shops or on the Internet, and are a good investment.

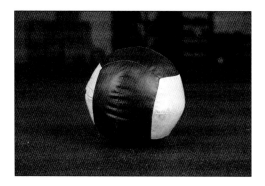

Exercise Step

For some of the exercises, it is useful to have a step or platform that can be used to make the movement easier. For example, the push-up type exercises can be made easier if the hands are raised relative to the feet, as the lower body is supporting more body weight. Most gyms will have steps of varying heights, or otherwise have graduated blocks that can be used to modify the height of the step as needed.

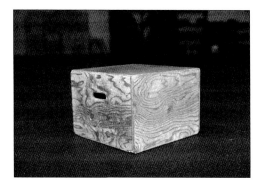

If you do not belong to a gym, you can purchase exercise steps and platforms on the Internet or in good sports shops for home use. In addition, you can also use objects around the home, such as stairs, steps or even the edges of sofas. Be creative, but always safe.

Barbell

A piece of equipment needed for the shoulder dislocate exercise and some other movements is the barbell. It should preferably be light and strong, and suitable for small weights. Steer clear of the Olympic-style barbell, as the bar alone weighs 20kg (44lb) and is therefore not very useful for the vast majority of readers.

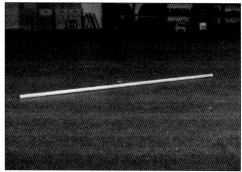

The ideal barbell to use would be the same as the one used in group exercise classes. These are usually much shorter and lighter than full-size Olympic barbells, and accommodate small weights easily, making them perfect for the exercises we advocate in this book. You may even find that a wooden dowel, such as a broom handle, is sufficient and provides a low-cost and accessible alternative.

Elastic Therapy Band

The elastic therapy band can be very useful when it comes to body-weight exercise. In this book we use it for some of the shoulder movements, such as the shoulder dislocate alternative. Elastic therapy bands for exercise come in many different strengths and

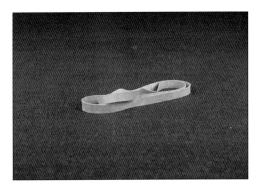

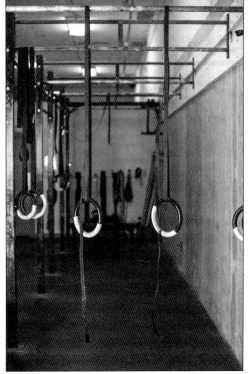

thicknesses, with some being very easy to stretch and others providing more resistance. Most gyms will have bands of varying strengths. If you are not a member of a gym, or if you train at home, elastic therapy bands can be found at low cost on the Internet or in good sports shops.

Gymnastic Rings

Gymnastic rings are perhaps the most specialised piece of equipment that can be used in this book. We do not suggest many exercises requiring this apparatus; however, if you like body-weight exercise, gymnastic rings are generally a useful thing to have. They are seldom seen in most commercial gyms, but the benefits of using them are undisputed. Gymnasts are widely regarded as being some of the strongest athletes (kg for kg) on earth, and so anything that can be taken from their training methodology and used in injury prevention and rehabilitation is well worth it.

As gymnastic rings are not commonly available in gyms, you will probably have to purchase some. They are actually quite cheap if you buy the nylon versions (rather than the official wooden rings), and they will last a lifetime if properly looked after. Rings come with straps that can be used to attach them to a pull-up bar or other fastenings. It is a good idea to make sure that this secure point is sufficiently high, preferably above head height. This way, you will be able to lower the rings to floor level or waist level and have plenty of space above to move. This is especially true with exercises such as the German hang (Chapter 5, Goal Exercise 5.14), where you need to be suspended in the air while close to the ground.

4

The Role of Nutrition and Recovery

A significant part of injury prevention and rehabilitation is knowing when to rest. Contrary to what many people believe, the body does not get stronger and more resilient during training sessions or workouts. The body repairs itself when it gets the chance, and this occurs when you engage in rest. The meaning of rest here is not necessarily a day on which you do absolutely nothing, but a day on which you perform no excessive or repeated physical activity. This 'rest' day will give the body a chance to recuperate and repair the damage done to it in the training sessions you have performed.

In this chapter we are going to look at various factors regarding nutrition, rest and recovery that are important to consider for injury resilience and rehabilitation.

▪ Nutrition

There is an old saying along the lines of 'you cannot out-train a bad diet'. This suggests that all of the physical activity in the world will struggle to outweigh the effects of a poor or inadequate diet. For this reason, we cannot ignore the importance of this subject when

developing a book on physical training. Your time is precious and we want you to maximise the gains from your hard work and efforts.

In addition to rest and good-quality sleep, nutrition is a key factor in recovering from workouts, staying injury free and rehabilitating existing injuries. There are two factors that must be considered when talking about nutrition: the first is the type or quality of nutrient, and the second is quantity. It may be obvious that meat, fish, eggs, vegetables, fruit and other natural foods are the types that you should eat. Natural, unprocessed foods present the body with easy-to-access nutrients in a form that our digestive systems have evolved to deal with.

It is a little trickier, however, to quantify the amount or volume of food that should be consumed to recover and grow following workouts, and to reduce the onset of chronic musculoskeletal injury. On the one hand, you must eat enough food so as to not deprive the body of the nutrients that it needs, but not so much that unwanted weight gain becomes an issue. Thankfully, it is very difficult to eat so much natural food that non-lean weight gain results. Even the largest and strongest humans on the planet (athletes who compete in professional strongman competitions) have to force themselves to eat huge quantities of food to get as big as they are. Natural food is rarely high in calories, and so mountains of vegetables will still only contain a similar calorie content to a very small portion of junk food. Junk food tends to be 'dense' in calories, and so to eat enough of it to fill you up means consuming a large amount of energy. And do not even get us started on washing it down with a fizzy or juice drink. Such foods and drinks are often high in sugars and/or saturated fats. It is now accepted that a calorie is not just a calorie: the source of that unit of energy is important to understand, as some chemicals are processed much more easily than others, while some go straight to storage (usually as fat).

The quantity of food that you need will vary depending on a number of factors, including age, height, weight, muscle mass, training history and genetics. We can only offer general guidelines here, since every reader will differ with respect to the factors listed above. The first guideline is to eat at least three meals a day, ideally spaced out equally. You do not want to get into the habit of missing meals or of eating a small amount at one sitting and then a large amount at another.

The second guideline is to ensure that a protein source is present in every meal. Protein is the nutrient that has the highest satiety rating of any nutrient, keeping you feeling fuller for longer. Protein also provides the building blocks of muscle and connective tissues, such as tendons and ligaments; these are all structures stressed and strained by physical training and daily postures and movements. Developing lean mass in the form of muscle will raise your resting metabolism, meaning that even

at rest you will have energy-hungry cells that require feeding; this will contribute to keeping your weight under control. It also means that you must keep feeding the beast in order to maintain that newly gained muscle mass. Having well-developed muscles and connective tissues will also contribute to your physical resilience by protecting joints and absorbing external and internal forces.

The third guideline is to make sure that you drink enough water during the day. Chronic dehydration can be misinterpreted by the brain as hunger, driving the desire to take on unneeded calories instead of essential fluids. Muscle, connective tissue and joints require an adequate water composition to ensure normal physiological functioning and resistance to daily trauma.

Avoid junk and processed food wherever possible for the reasons discussed above. As a simple clarification, junk and processed food is anything that is far from the natural source food. This includes all of the usual culprits, such as fast food, sugary snacks, drinks that are a luminous colour, and anything else with an unnatural appearance. You can also add to this list processed sugar and flour, and any other product that has been highly refined or processed.

Basic Nutrition for Growth and Repair

While the advice so far in this chapter has been general enough to improve health for the vast majority of people, there are some specific nutrients that will help with injury prevention and rehabilitation.

Protein

You are made of protein. From the enzymes that regulate your cell activity, to the structural muscle and connective tissue fibres, protein is essential for repairing and replacing such things on a daily basis. As the entire premise of this book revolves around building resilience and strength in the body to reduce the incidence and severity of injury, and to rehabilitate existing injuries, it makes sense that protein is perhaps number one on the list of important nutrients. The protein that you consume in your diet, whether it is from animal or plant sources, is made up of building blocks called *amino acids*. Once digested, the amino acid 'blocks' are reorganised to build new structures within your body. This process could be the repair of the ligament collagen fibres that you damaged during an ankle sprain; it could also mean an increase in muscle mass to support and power occupational or sporting activities. With regard to building muscle mass, or at least ensuring adequate muscle repair, the general daily recommendation is to take in two grams of dietary protein for every kilogram of body weight.

Calcium

Strong bones are essential for maintaining skeletal strength and for protecting against bony injury, such as a stress fracture. Calcium is needed for strong bones, as it is one of the key minerals that impregnates and hardens the protein framework of your skeleton. This particular nutrient is often linked solely to a dairy-based diet, but there are in fact many dietary sources of calcium. Lots of people, not necessarily just those who are lactose intolerant, are moving towards a dairy-free diet. By learning about other sources of calcium, you need never be short on this essential mineral nutrient, whatever your preference. Sources of calcium include:

- Milk
- Kale
- Sardines
- Yogurt
- Broccoli
- Watercress
- Cheese
- Bok Choy

Vitamin D

Vitamin D is a nutrient that is tied inextricably to calcium, in that the body needs vitamin D to be able to process calcium for bone health. In other words, you can drink all of the milk in the world, but if you do not ingest adequate vitamin D, your body will not be able to utilise all of the calcium.

Vitamin D can be found in a range of foods, and a balanced diet should provide sufficient amounts. The body will also synthesise vitamin D with exposure to sunlight, but the vitamin is more readily available from sunshine, with the consensus being around 20 minutes of direct sunshine a day. This does not mean exposure to harmful UV rays, and so sunscreen should still be used. Exercising outdoors for 20 minutes a day with a bulletproof-body routine will contribute immensely to physical health and resilience.

Vitamin C

Most of us have heard the old adage that vitamin C is good for keeping colds away, but the evidence for this is lacking. What most people are not aware of is that vitamin C is also very good for injury prevention and rehabilitation. There are a number of reasons for this:

1. It helps in the building of collagen, which is vital for repairing connective tissues, such as ligaments and tendons, and the general support structures of the body.
2. It increases the amount of iron absorbed from food, useful in

haemoglobin production for improved oxygen-carrying capacity.

3. It is a known antioxidant, protecting the body's cells from harmful free-radical activity.

There are a lot of foods that contain vitamin C – here are a few suggestions:

- Broccoli
- Papaya
- Bell peppers
- Brussels sprouts
- Strawberries
- Pineapple
- Oranges
- Kiwi fruit
- Cauliflower
- Grapefruit
- Tomatoes

How much vitamin C to include in your diet is up for debate: the normal recommended daily allowance is 90mg for men and 75mg for women. Some studies have suggested that increasing this amount to 400mg can be more optimal for health. One scientific study recommended taking 1,000–2,000mg of vitamin C every day for a short time (five days) following injury. Vitamin C is water soluble, however, and cannot be stored in the body; it is therefore likely that excessive amounts will be lost without any benefit.

Before you run off to the shops to buy hundreds of vitamin C pills, we offer a word of caution. Massively increasing vitamin C intake can result in some side effects, including nausea, abdominal cramps, headaches, fatigue and even kidney stones.

The Importance of Carbohydrate

Carbohydrate has had some bad press recently regarding health and weight loss.

The media can have a tendency to advocate 'throwing the baby out with the bath water'; with respect to diet, this means excluding even beneficial carbohydrate. Carbohydrate is an important nutrient that contributes to health and athletic performance. What we really need to be aware of is the *source* of the carbohydrates being taken into the body.

We can understand this a little more easily if we think of starchy and non-starchy carbohydrates. *Non-starchy carbohydrates* are those that still provide the energy that our bodies need, but do not have the high calorie content or the blood-sugar raising properties that starchy carbohydrates do. Leafy vegetables, carrots, cauliflower, green beans, sweet corn and sweet potatoes are some examples of non-starchy vegetables. Try to include as many of these foods as possible in your diet. A typical meal, for example, might be grilled chicken breast, peas, broccoli, carrots and brown rice. This will contain protein from the chicken, fat from the chicken, and non-starchy carbohydrates from the vegetables. Everything the body needs will be present in this type of meal, and as long as you try to stick to this type of eating plan, you will find that your health, weight-loss, fitness and injury-prevention goals will be achieved.

In contrast, *starchy carbohydrates* are those that are found, for example, in bread, pasta, potatoes and rice. They are normally stodgy and moderate to high in calorie content, and can contribute to weight gain if eaten to excess. If we expand this to include processed foods, such as cakes, donuts, ice cream and chocolate, you can see how eating these might contribute to weight gain and to an increase in body fat percentage. It makes sense from a health perspective to limit the intake of these types of food as much as possible. Eating rice and potatoes is fine, but try to go for brown rice, and limit potatoes to a sensible minimum.

The real culprit is processed and refined carbohydrate. As the name suggests, these are not naturally occurring states of carbohydrate; they are, however, derived from natural foods, and this is where the confusion can arise. You may often see products being badged as 'no added sugar', or 'contains natural sugars'. Sugar is a natural substance, found in abundance throughout many natural foods. It is the way in which this sugar is delivered to the body, however, that requires attention. Some sugars after being processed are difficult for the body to handle, and so either are converted to storage (weight gain!), or add to the workload of the liver (where toxins are processed!).

Across the developed world, we are now seeing an increase in metabolic syndromes, obesity and non-alcoholic liver disease. Further discussion on this topic is beyond the scope of this book, but there are plenty of other information sources out there from which you can learn more. A final word on this matter – make your body work for its calories. If they come easily, and in large amounts, then common sense might suggest this is not what our systems have evolved to process.

Hydration

The statistic that says that the human body is composed of 60% water indicates that this often-overlooked nutrient is essential, and that this is one fact worth taking seriously. Chronic dehydration is thought to affect a significant percentage of the population; the situation is made worse by the modern diet, as many people substitute other drinks for water. Relying on coffee, tea, soft drinks and possibly alcohol as a source of hydration is an unwise decision. Both coffee and tea contain caffeine, which is a known diuretic, and this will cause you to lose water by urinating more. Soft drinks contain water, but they also contain a concoction of other chemicals that you may not want in your body, including copious amounts of refined and processed sugar. In addition to being 'empty' calories that cannot really help to repair your body, sugar will make losing weight (if this is one of your goals) much more difficult. There really is no point in moving one step forwards if your regular soft drink intake is moving you two steps backwards.

Many people face the problem of not knowing how much water to drink in a given time period. To help you out in this regard, we have included a simple table to show you how much water you should aim to drink in a 24-hour period (Table 4.1). Note that the water intake will vary, depending on a number of factors, including climate, fitness, body size and the amount of exercise performed.

Alcohol Consumption

Alcohol consumption is a debatable issue in terms of its effect on health, with several reports suggesting that moderate intake, such as a glass of red wine, can actually be beneficial. If this is the case, the benefits are unlikely to be entirely derived from the alcohol, but rather from the properties of the grapes that make up the wine.

If you are injured or rehabilitating an injury, or perhaps seeking to stay injury free, the best course of action would be to drink as little alcohol as possible. Processing alcohol requires time and effort, and incurs a cost to your body in terms of energy and nutrition that cannot be used for growth and repair to build a stronger and more resilient body. If you have an acute injury, be aware that

■ Table 4.1. Recommended water intake (24-hour period).

Your weight (kg)	Your weight (lb)	Water intake in litres
45.5	100	1.5
50	110	1.7
54.5	120	1.8
59	130	2
64	140	2.1
68	150	2.3
73	160	2.4
77	170	2.6
82	180	2.7
86	190	2.9
91	200	3
95.5	210	3.2
100	220	3.3
104.5	230	3.5
109	240	3.6
113.5	250	3.8
118	260	3.9
122.5	270	4.1
127	280	4.2
132	290	4.4
136.5	300	4.5

alcohol acts as a vasodilator (causes dilation of the walls of blood vessels), and may cause further swelling in the injured area; this may in turn increase the time to heal.

■ Rest and Recovery

Sleep

Sufficient good-quality sleep is a fundamental aspect of injury prevention and rehabilitation. Getting enough sleep is vital in order for the body to repair itself properly, but a lack of it is unfortunately rife in today's modern culture; reasons for this may include worrying about work, family, money or health. Sleep deprivation may reduce your ability to cope with these factors during your waking hours and so lead to a vicious circle. Talk through your problems before you try to sleep, or even write down your problems before bed in an attempt to offload your mind.

In addition to the normal worries of life causing below-par sleep quality and quantity, poor 'sleep hygiene' is now well recognised as a modern-day affliction. Sleep hygiene refers to daily habits that can be modified to enable better sleep. Going to bed at a sensible time and not staying up to watch television can improve the quality of sleep immensely. Go to bed when you start feeling tired, rather than fighting the urge and distracting yourself with other activities, such as watching TV or sitting at a computer.

Avoid using display-screen technology, such as your phone or tablet, before going to sleep. It is common in the modern world for many people to check their phones or electronic devices before they go to bed, or even to peruse them while in bed. Reading in bed is increasingly being carried out using electronic devices, much to the detriment of getting to sleep successfully. There are now filters and specific modes on many devices that reduce the blue light that is known to impact on brain function. If you have to use your electronic device in bed, it is a good idea to turn the filter feature on, or better still leave your phone in another room. Your social media notifications will not go anywhere, and will be waiting for you in the morning.

Ensuring that you are in bed before midnight is often regarded as sound sleeping advice; this is especially true if you have to get up early. The notion of eight hours of solid sleep has recently been questioned, with some scientists suggesting that the body naturally wakes after three to four hours, before later needing a further block of three to four hours. Just do not eat biscuits during the break!

The power nap has also gained popularity in recent years, and science is beginning to support this practice. The body seems to have a natural dip in the mid-afternoon that supports a power nap. There are also recommendations to consume caffeine before the power nap to improve post-nap alertness.

Quality sleep regulates normal hormone control, including growth and stress hormones, as well as the hormones involved in blood-sugar control. The effects of improving your sleep may therefore have an impact on many areas of your life, including psychological wellbeing, weight control and physical resilience to injury.

Reducing Stress

Reducing stress is another important aspect of injury prevention. Stress, in whatever forms it takes, can have profound detrimental effects on the body. Psychological stress is difficult to avoid in the modern world; worries about money, work, the pressures of family and the uncertainty of the future can all be very real. Unless measures are taken to deal with the thoughts associated with these perceived problems, the stress that results can soon spiral out of control. This stress can manifest itself in the form of physical problems, from raised blood pressure to increased muscle tension. Chapter 5 of this book examines how stress can show itself in shoulder and neck posture, later leading to dysfunction. You may be familiar with the sensation of increased shoulder/neck muscle tension causing aches and pains.

A discussion of the ways of dealing with daily issues and life in general is not within the

scope of this book, but there are a few things that you can do to help combat the rise of stress and its impact on the body. First, make sure that you remain active, both physically and mentally; a strong body and mind will make coping with stressful situations much easier. Second, ensure that your sleep and nutrition are optimal, as described earlier. Eating well will give you more energy, a better physical composition and better health in general, all of which will help deal with stress; they may even resolve some of the health and weight issues that caused the stress in the first place.

How you spend your rest days is also very important. If you have a perceived stressful job and life, then find positive ways to use this stress response, such as exercise or an active hobby. Rest and relax during the days that you are away from work. Be with people whose company you enjoy, and surround yourself with positive distractions.

Ways of Sitting

Many desk-based jobs require sitting down for long periods of time; this can contribute towards many of the physical problems explored throughout this book. Tight or weak muscles may eventually manifest themselves in chronic injury and pain that niggle away at you during day-to-day activities. Two of the most common consequences of sitting for long periods are shortened hamstrings and spinal problems, especially in the area of the lumbar spine.

If your job requires you to sit at a desk, there are things you can do to make this less of a problem: getting up and stretching the hamstrings, hips and spine every hour is good practice. Look through the relevant chapters of this book and add some simple mobility exercises to your working day (if space and company policy allow). You might also try working at a standing desk, as this may negate the constant stress of a sitting posture. If your place of work has an ergonomic assessment facility, we recommend that you use it. If it does not, ask yourself if your work set-up or postures feel right to you. If they don't feel right, they probably aren't, and so play around with them.

At home you may also find that you spend a lot of time sitting; this may be for a number of reasons, including watching television, reading, eating an evening meal or even spending time with family or friends. There are some adjustments that can be made here, though, with perhaps the best solution being to sit on the floor with the legs stretched out in front. Even a cross-legged position on the floor will provide a welcome stretch to the hips and lower back. These positions might be uncomfortable at first (especially if your hamstrings and lower back are tight); however, soon enough your hamstrings will lengthen and become more flexible, and the positions will become much more comfortable. Sitting like this will not require any special equipment, and the normal activities you perform at home can still be enjoyed with little or no impact. Even better, try doing some of these activities without sitting at all; for example, spend time catching up with family by going for a walk with them, or read while standing up.

Forward Head Posture

A physical ailment that has appeared in recent years is the forward head posture: in this condition the head and neck jut forwards, leading to muscle imbalances in the neck and shoulders. A common cause of this problem is the use of mobile phones and other electronic screen devices, whereby the head is constantly looking down and fixed in a restricted field

of vision for extended periods. The long-term consequences of this are not yet clear, as such electronic screen devices have not been around long enough for firm conclusions to be drawn.

The weight of the head is approximately 5–6kg (11–13lb). If the head and the shoulders move forwards, out of ideal alignment, the activation of the neck extensor muscles will increase dramatically. For every 2.5cm (1″) of forward head posture, the weight of the head on the spine can increase by approximately 4.5kg (10lb); this may lead to increased neck muscle tension and excessive strain on the underlying joints of the neck.

To combat forward head posture, the best course of action is to limit the use of mobiles and other electronic devices as much as possible; at the very least, one should try to use them in a way that will not contribute towards the problem. Ask yourself whether or not using a device like this is contributing towards your day. If checking social media is not impacting your life in a positive way, and is adding to the development of a forward head posture, then put the device down and start moving.

Chapter 11 of this book covers some simple and effective exercises to supplement this advice and reduce that forward head posture.

Overtraining

In the context of injury prevention and rehabilitation, the concept of overtraining is worth considering. In its simplest definition, *overtraining* refers to the act of training with too much intensity and too often, with inadequate rest between training sessions, leading to reduced training gains; in other words, more becomes less. This type of training causes many physical and psychological problems, but the main one that we will consider here is the impact of a lack of adequate recovery. If you train too often at a high intensity, the physical trauma that is done to the body will not be repaired before the next training session. If the sessions keep on coming at the same intensity and frequency, the body will slowly deteriorate until a point where injuries become inevitable and overall physical performance decreases. Such relentless stress on the body will reduce the resilience of bone, muscle and connective tissues (such as ligaments and tendons)

to further stress. You may also experience mental fatigue and adverse effects on your immune and hormonal systems.

To deal with the issue of overtraining, it is best to keep a training log and note down when you feel tired or worn out, or when you start to get niggling injures. If you are an endurance sport athlete, try training with a heart rate monitor and log your efforts. These methods can be very effective for identifying the onset of overtraining and knowing when to take a step back. Sometimes, less is more!

5

The Shoulder

◼ Introduction to the Shoulder

You may know the shoulder as a single joint that is capable of an amazing range of movements and functions. In reality, it is best considered as a *complex*. This term is not used because it is a complicated joint, but rather to highlight the fact that there is an orchestra of components all working together to bring about movement and stability of the shoulder region. The shoulder has allowed humans to interact with, and manipulate, the external world. From washing your hair to fastening a bra, the shoulder is called upon to move through a range not seen in any other joint; in sport and exercise these demands increase significantly.

Humans display an emotional connection with the shoulder joint. Notice how the shoulders can rise upwards towards the ears during times of stress, with an uncomfortable tension building up in the surrounding muscles. The shoulder complex can also reflect our mood – the slumped shoulders when we are feeling low or the shoulders pulled back with pride. When painful, the shoulder has an ability that no other joint

seems to have to the same degree; it can immobilise itself. Picture the fallen Tour de France rider cradling their immobilised arm after a collarbone (clavicle) injury. It is not unusual to see a patient with a frozen shoulder reaching across their body to grip their painful upper arm and fix it against their body. In this way it can be totally relieved of its functional duties.

By acknowledging the shoulder complex for what it is – a collection of moving and stabilising parts – you will better appreciate the overview of anatomy that follows. This will lead you on to discover how and why some of these structures become dysfunctional, causing pain and restriction of movement.

◼ Functional Anatomy of the Shoulder

Passive Structures

The term *passive structures* will be used in its very broadest sense throughout this book to refer to any structure in the musculoskeletal system that cannot move itself. That is, its resting state can only be changed by something acting upon it, whether this is gravity, somebody moving it on a person's behalf, or a muscle and tendon pulling against it.

The passive, or inert, structures are those that give the fundamental shape and inherent stability to the joint; examples are bones, cartilage, ligaments, capsules and bursae. The relationship of these structures can be seen in Figure 5.1.

The obvious bones of the shoulder complex are the scapula, humerus and clavicle. We should also include the posterior chest wall created by the ribs, and the upper breast bone (sternum).

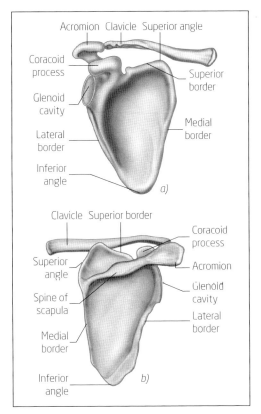

■ **Figure 5.1.** Bones of the shoulder complex: (a) anterior view; (b) posterior view.

> **KEY POINT** *The joint between the clavicle and sternum (sternoclavicular joint) is the only true joint connecting the arm to the rest of the body!*
> *It is a small joint with a tremendous responsibility.*

The sternoclavicular joint does not act alone in providing attachment and transmitting forces between the body and the arm. When performing body-weight exercise, or any form of physical loading, there is a special relationship between the scapula and ribcage that creates a powerful bridge for the passage of power. It is not considered a true articulation, yet this 'false' joint is key to the proper functioning, positioning and stability of the shoulder joint. Dysfunction of this relationship can lead to multiple pain problems around the shoulder complex and can cause some of the problems explored below. As you will discover later in this chapter, body-weight exercises are ideally suited to addressing many of the problems arising from poor scapulothoracic movement control.

The shoulder complex is reinforced by ligaments and a joint capsule. These structures stabilise the moving parts of the shoulder, limit excessive or unwanted movements and provide positional feedback to your brain. The *subdeltoid bursa* seen in Figure 5.2 is so named because of its location beneath the deltoid muscle of the shoulder.

The subdeltoid bursa is also referred to as the *subacromial bursa* because it partially sits under the bony shelf of the scapula, known as the *acromion*. It is here that this fluid-filled sack becomes dysfunctional and a potential source of shoulder pain (see 'Subacromial Pain Syndrome' below).

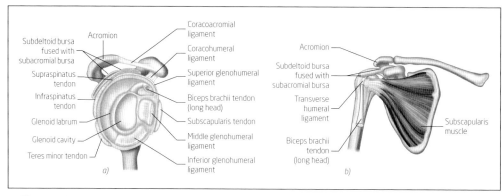

■ **Figure 5.2.** The subdeltoid bursa: (a) right arm, lateral view; (b) right arm, anterior view (cut).

Active Structures

In their simplest form, *active (contracting) structures* will be regarded here as those capable of generating movement. Muscles do this by contracting (shortening) in response to electrical impulses generated either consciously or subconsciously. As they contract, they pull on their tendons, which in turn exert a force on bone to cause movement at a joint. Because muscles can only pull and not push, they cannot return a joint to its original position where gravity or other forces are neutralised. You will therefore see muscles arranged in opposing pairs; perhaps the most famous of these duos crosses both the shoulder and the elbow – the biceps and triceps – as shown in Figure 5.3.

If you are asked to think of other muscles at the shoulder, your first thought might be the deltoid muscle. While this muscle is absolutely essential in generating force at the shoulder to power the arm from the side or to press it above the head, it actually has a very minor role in rehabilitating the shoulder.

KEY POINT *For bulletproof shoulders, focus on developing the muscles and tendons of the rotator cuff, and the muscles that control the scapula.*

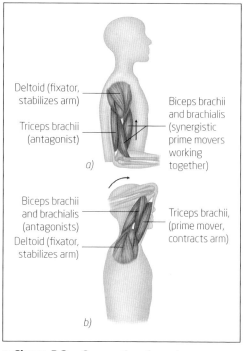

■ **Figure 5.3.** Group action of muscles: (a) flexing the arm at the elbow; (b) extending the arm at the elbow.

The *rotator cuff* is a dynamic compressive support that maintains the head of the upper arm bone (humerus) in the socket provided by the scapula. It plays a very important role in shoulder joint function. In addition to being dynamic stabilisers, the muscles and tendons of the rotator cuff contribute to proper movement

at the true shoulder (glenohumeral) joint.
The rotator cuff is made up of:

- Supraspinatus
- Infraspinatus
- Subscapularis
- Teres minor

All four of these short muscles originate
from the scapula and insert on the head of
the humerus. If the position of these bones
relative to one another is altered through poor

posture or muscle imbalance, the function of
the cuff muscles will be compromised.

We must, however, consider all the muscles
acting on the scapula if we truly wish to
rehabilitate or make resilient the shoulder
complex. These muscles include the trapezius,
rhomboids, levator scapulae, latissimus
dorsi, teres major, deltoid, pectoralis
major, pectoralis minor, serratus anterior,
coracobrachialis, biceps brachii and triceps
brachii. Isolating these muscles and their
functions would be difficult and possibly
counterproductive. Functional loading will
therefore recruit these muscles as and when
required to perform the movement properly.
This is the basis of body-weight exercise as a
rehabilitation/physical resilience method.

> **KEY POINT** *The body recruits groups of
> muscles to perform a particular function
> rather than individual muscles.*

■ Common Shoulder Dysfunction

The wide variety of pure movements normally
available at the glenohumeral joint combine
to create an extensive circular movement,
known as *circumduction*. This can be fully
appreciated when you 'windmill' your arms.
The large degree of movement is facilitated
by the scapula as it travels over the posterior
ribcage. To fully maximise shoulder function,
we therefore also need to consider the
position of the ribcage, as this is the 'stage'
on which the shoulder joint performs.
If this is poorly positioned because of posture
or trauma, then stress is placed on other
structures to compensate.

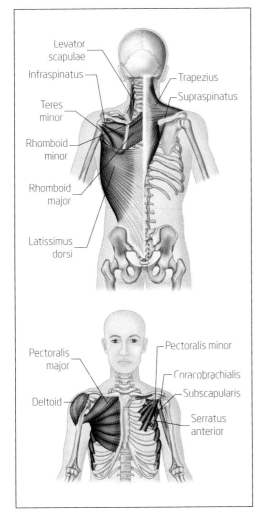

■ **Figure 5.4.** Rotator cuff muscles and the
muscles attaching the upper limb to the trunk.

During a diagnosis of dysfunction at the
shoulder, you may hear nonspecific terms

such as *impingement syndrome* or *frozen shoulder*. Paradoxically, the better our understanding of pathology has become, the looser and more nondescript the diagnoses have been in recent years. This actually reflects a better understanding of shoulder problems – tissue dysfunctions often coexist! It is very difficult to pinpoint the cause of shoulder pain to a single structure, and there has not been a scan invented that can detect pain. Dysfunction, on the other hand, can be obvious to a well-trained health or medical professional. The shoulder is a fairly honest joint that often reveals its secrets through patterns of pain and movement.

Some of the key features of common shoulder problems will be explored next.

Subacromial Pain Syndrome

You may hear this condition described as *impingement syndrome, rotator cuff disease* or even *rotator cuff tendinopathy*. It is thought to be caused by an entrapment of the soft tissues in the space below the bony shelf of the acromion, hence the term *subacromial* (Figure 5.5). This rotator cuff dysfunction may in turn lead to reduced control of the head of the humerus bone and contribute further to the subacromial impingement.

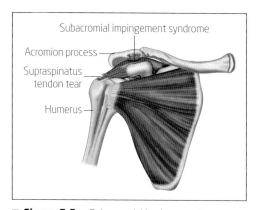

Subacromial impingement syndrome

Acromion process

Supraspinatus tendon tear

Humerus

■ **Figure 5.5.** Subacromial impingement.

In clinical practice and in the research literature, the term *subacromial pain syndrome* is becoming more common. This is partly because it is difficult to observe impingement on scans like ultrasound, but also because we cannot be sure of a single structure being the cause of pain. The 'impingement' may involve not just the rotator cuff tendons but also the long head of the biceps muscle and the bursa. Thickening of the bursa, the rotator cuff tendons and the shoulder ligaments can further reduce the available space for movement. Add in poor shoulder posture and you have a recipe for pain. According to some research, subacromial impingement syndrome is the most common diagnosis for shoulder pain.

Before we leave the overview of this pathology, it is worth considering the concept of tendinopathy of the rotator cuff tendons. It has often been regarded as an 'overuse' tendon disorder, but this has been brought into question more recently. Some evidence suggests that degenerative tendon change is due to many factors, one of which could be a form of underuse; that means not used sufficiently in the context in which the injury may have occurred. This again suggests that loading the tendon in a controlled way with body-weight exercises may make the tendon more robust and restore pain-free function.

Very often, small tears may be found in the rotator cuff tendons; however, these are often treated effectively with nothing more than physiotherapy/loading exercise and modified shoulder movements. The tears may respond well to steroid injections, but this is considered to potentially weaken the tendon further and possibly increase the risk of further tears or rupture. If you are unsure, seek advice from your qualified medical or health professional.

KEY EXERCISE 5.1: SCAPULA DIP

Primary Target Area: Muscles around the scapulae

Sets: 3
Reps: 10
Rest: 30–45 seconds

LEVEL 3

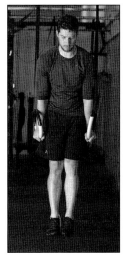 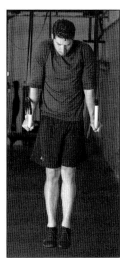

This is an exercise for activating the scapula muscles; it uses the same starting position as a triceps dip, but has no movement from the elbows. The scapula dip is a useful exercise for those who are not used to supporting the entirety of their own body weight. You will need access to a dip bar as described in the equipment chapter, or other similar set-up. If you have a kitchen worktop that meets in an internal corner, you may find this a suitable surface for this exercise.

1. To perform the scapula dip, grab the dip bar with both hands facing inwards. Push yourself up until your elbows are straight.
2. From here, draw your shoulder blades downwards, away from your ears, without bending your elbows. Keep going until you cannot rise any further. This is the starting position.
3. Lower yourself down without bending your elbows. It should feel like your ears are dropping to meet your shoulders.
4. Push back up again until you reach the starting position. This counts as one repetition.

Teaching Points

The scapula dip is tough not primarily because of the strength required, but because many people struggle to keep their elbows straight when performing the movement. Try to isolate the shoulders as much as possible, and think about keeping the elbows straight to avoid excessive muscular strain here. Watching yourself in a mirror or getting a training partner to help is a good idea.

Rotator Cuff Injury

Much of the discussion on this topic has already been covered in the previous account of subacromial pain syndrome. In many cases, traumatic tears to the rotator cuff tendons will be small or only penetrate part way through the thickness of the tendon. Movement-based rehabilitation, with or without steroid injection, is often tried in the first instance. This is where your body-weight rehabilitation program can provide good functional recovery. However, where there has been more severe trauma, or perhaps your tendons are not what they were 60 years ago, you may want to get a thorough assessment from a qualified and experienced health or medical professional. If they do suspect a large tear or rupture of the rotator cuff tendons, you may be referred for a scan of the shoulder. Even in these cases, surgery may not be the best option, and you may be advised to initially try movement-based interventions. You may choose to slowly introduce body-weight exercises into your routine as pain and function allow.

KEY EXERCISE 5.2: FROG STANCE

Target Area: Muscles around the scapulae
Sets: 3
Duration: Hold for 10–20 seconds, once in position
Rest: 30–45 seconds

LEVEL 3

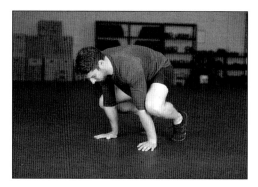

The frog stance, also called the *elephant stand* or *crane*, is a static strength position used mainly in yoga and gymnastics. It is valued for its ability to build strength in the upper body, especially the shoulder complex, forearms and hands. The frog stance has an element of balance to it; therefore, when performing it, make sure that the surrounding area is free of objects. We recommend using an exercise mat to protect against any falls.

1. To perform the frog stance, crouch down and place your hands on the floor, shoulder-width apart. Splay your fingers wide to aid in control and balance.

2. Place your knees on the outsides of your elbows, allowing the arms to take some of your body weight.

3. Lean forwards, moving more and more weight onto the arms. Allow the elbows to bend if they want to. Hold at this point if you feel you are not able to take any more weight through the arms. As you get stronger over the weeks, you can progress the exercise as described in steps 4–5.

4. Keep leaning forwards, moving onto the tips of the toes. Once you get into this position, you will feel as though the upper body is supporting most of your body weight. From here, try to raise your feet into the air slightly so that only your hands are in contact with the ground.

5. Hold this position for as long as possible, using the muscles in the hands and forearms to control your balance. Keep your shoulder blades down, away from your ears!

Teaching Points

The frog stance is not overly difficult strengthwise, but the main issue for many people is wrist flexibility and the balance aspect of the movement. See the exercises in Chapter 7 to improve your wrist strength.

To improve your balance, there is no substitute for practice. Accordingly, make this exercise a regular part of your physical routine, and you will soon see rapid progress.

Stiff, or 'Frozen', Shoulder

The term *frozen shoulder* is commonly used in public parlance to describe a stiff and painful shoulder of any origin. Clinically, the term has been criticised, as it does not describe the exact condition. The current trend is to call it a *contracted shoulder*, and this in part suggests that the capsule around the true shoulder joint has become tight or shrunken. This condition reduces movement in the same way that a very tight and shrunken jumper would limit your arm movements.

Frozen shoulders are generally regarded as being of two types, depending on whether the condition happened for no apparent reason (primary), or whether there was a recent history of trauma or immobilisation of the shoulder (secondary). Crudely speaking, the condition is considered to go through a freezing stage, a frozen stage and a thawing stage. The first stage is characterised by increasing pain and stiffness, and this can really begin to disturb your sleep and daily function. The middle stage involves a levelling-off of symptoms, and you coming to terms with the restriction. The final phase sees the shoulder become progressively more mobile and less painful. The literature varies in its views about recovery rates, but most frozen shoulders will recover almost all function in one to three years.

It is recommended to exercise caution with any sort of physical rehabilitation for this condition. In the early stages, exercise is less likely to work and could cause a flare-up of your pain. The body-weight routines proposed here are better suited to the latter stages of the condition, but should only be performed if the joint can move into the required positions. As the frozen shoulder progresses through the different stages, so too can your body-weight exercises.

KEY EXERCISE 5.3: CHEST STRETCH

Target Area: Shoulders, chest
Sets: 3
Duration: Hold for 15 seconds
Rest: 10 seconds   **LEVEL 1**

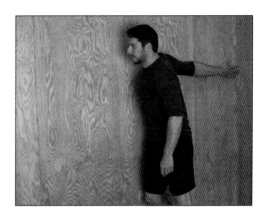

The pectoral muscles of the chest can have a large impact on the flexibility of the shoulders, especially in bringing the arms over the head and in moving the arms back horizontally. The muscles can pull the shoulder into a rounded position. Being able to move the shoulders without hindrance is therefore important in order to maintain optimal function and stay injury free.

1. To perform the chest stretch, place one palm against a solid object, such as a wall or doorframe. Make sure that your hand is at the same level as your shoulders.
2. Keeping your elbow straight, turn your body in the opposite direction so that your chest opens.
3. Keep turning until you feel the stretch in your chest. Hold this position for the required time, change arms and repeat.

Teaching Points

As with most stretching, there comes a point when the level of your flexibility is sufficient to allow functional body movements. This process may take longer if you are recovering from a shoulder problem, such as the stiff shoulder, or if you have long-standing muscle shortening. From this point on, your stretching will take on a different purpose: for warming up and maintaining your level of flexibility. How long it takes will depend on many things, including your age, training background and initial flexibility.

Acromioclavicular Joint Dysfunction

The *acromioclavicular joint* is a small joint between the outer edge of the collarbone and the acromion part of the shoulder blade; it can be a source of discomfort and dysfunction. Problems may be precipitated by a trauma, such as falling onto an outstretched hand, or by a direct blow to the shoulder. In these cases, the injury can be classified in three degrees, with grade 1 being a mild sprain and grade 3 being disruption and dislocation of the joint. Grade 3 injuries are much less common, while grades 1 and 2 could benefit from some stability-focused body-weight exercises that target scapula and shoulder positioning and control.

In later life, the acromioclavicular joint may be affected by degenerative osteoarthritis. This can be the case particularly where there has been a history of heavy use or trauma in the affected shoulder. Here, the joint space has narrowed and the mechanics of the joint are not what they once were. Degenerative changes around the joint may even impact on the subacromial space, and so contribute to pain that is subacromial in origin (see above). Mobilising the joint through loaded body-weight exercise may be of benefit in this situation, but if you are unsure then seek initial advice from a suitably qualified and experienced health or medical professional.

KEY EXERCISE 5.4: BAND SHOULDER DISLOCATE

Primary Target Area: Shoulders, chest
Sets: 3
Reps: 10
Rest: 20 seconds

LEVEL 2

The band shoulder dislocate is the first of three variations of a shoulder mobility exercise. The words *shoulder dislocate* can conjure up a painful image, but it is nowhere near as excruciating as it sounds. It is a great exercise for increasing mobility in the shoulder joint.

For this band version, you will need an elastic therapy band to use as the resistance. This method allows the distance between the hands to be narrow or wide depending on the flexibility of the shoulders. Any elastic band

■ **Figure 5.6.** Acromioclavicular joint: (a) anterior view; (b) coronal view.

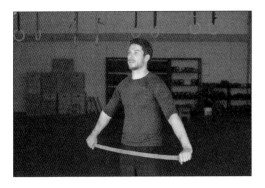

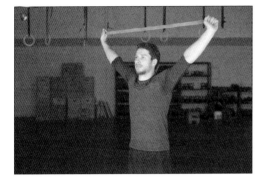

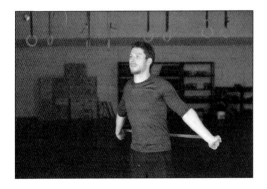

suited for exercise will work, and they can be found in gyms quite readily; they can also be purchased cheaply in sports shops and on the Internet.

1. To perform the band shoulder dislocate, grab an elastic band with both hands and hold it in front of your pelvis. Both elbows should be straight and your grip loose but strong.

2. How wide your hands are will dictate how tough the exercise will be: the wider your hands, the easier the movement, and the narrower your hands, the more difficult. The band will stretch if you need it to.

3. Start to raise the band up and over your head, keeping your elbows straight and your arms wide. As the band goes over your head, you will most likely feel tightness in the shoulders and need to widen the hands in order to reduce the pressure.

4. Keep going until the band reaches your lower back. At no point should you bend the elbows.

5. Reverse the movement until you reach the starting position. This counts as one repetition.

Teaching Points

Using the band for this first stage is very useful, as it allows you to widen your hands during the difficult parts and narrow them when it becomes easy. As you find the exercise becoming easier, you can start with your hands in a narrower position; this way, there will be more resistance when stretching the band as you move through the difficult phase of the movement.

Summary

Once you or your health/medical professional have come to a reasoned diagnosis, you can then start to plan your rehabilitation in the light of the expected timescale for recovery. The good news is that, given the nonspecific definitions of pathology at the shoulder, you need not concern yourself with specific isolated rehabilitation. Keep it functional, feasible, free from pain and, where possible, fun! The following section will guide you through some suggested body-weight exercises that can both prevent injury and promote recovery from injury of the shoulder complex.

■ Body-weight Exercises for Shoulder Injury Prevention and Rehabilitation

Now that you have an idea of the anatomy of the shoulder and some of the more common injuries that affect the area, it is time to look at body-weight exercises which will help to both prevent injury and rehabilitate existing injuries.

In general, the exercises are listed here in order of difficulty, with the easiest appearing first. Exercises that are similar, such as the scapula pull-up and the one-armed scapula pull-up, demonstrate how you can progress.

With regard to the difficulty of an exercise, we are talking about the strength and mobility required to perform it. Keep this in mind when trying to address your own rehabilitation or injury prevention goals.

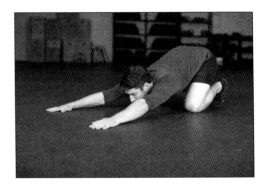

syndrome. This exercise is great for developing shoulder flexibility.

1. To perform the shoulder stretch, kneel down and place your palms flat against the floor in front of you.
2. Push your hips backwards and move your chest towards the ground. Keep pushing the shoulders and chest down to the ground to increase the stretch. Hold this for the required time and then rest.

Teaching Points
If you find that you can touch the ground with your chest, you can place your hands on a raised platform of some sort, such as a step or exercise box. This will allow you to stretch the shoulders further.

EXERCISE 5.5: SHOULDER STRETCH

Target Area: Shoulders, chest, back
Sets: 3
Duration: Hold for 15 seconds
Rest: 10 seconds   LEVEL 1

One excellent test of shoulder flexibility is the ability to raise the arms up over the head without any hindrance. This may be a limitation when recovering from a stiff shoulder, but may also be a predisposing factor for developing subacromial pain

EXERCISE 5.6: ROTATOR CUFF STRETCH

Primary Target Area: Rotator cuff muscles
Sets: 3
Duration: Hold for 10 seconds
Rest: 10 seconds   LEVEL 1

The rotator cuff musculature is a potential site of injury, as described previously. Stretching these muscles is challenging but very

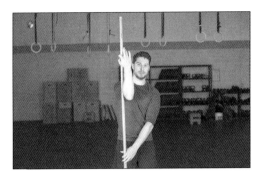

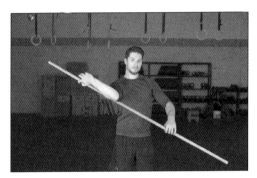

EXERCISE 5.7: SCAPULA FOAM ROLL

Primary Target Area: Muscles around the scapulae
Sets: 3
Duration: 10 seconds
Rest: 30–45 seconds

LEVEL 1

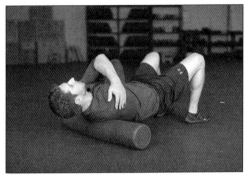

rewarding. This exercise will also stretch a stiff (frozen) shoulder, but go easy! You will need a bar for this stretch, the best option being either an exercise class barbell or a broom handle.

1. To stretch your rotator cuff, grasp a bar with one hand curled around, with the bar pressing against the outside of your upper arm.
2. With your free arm grab the bar towards the bottom, and pull it up towards the ceiling. You should feel a stretch deep in the shoulder. Hold this for 10 seconds, change arms and repeat.

Teaching Points

This stretch can feel strange at first, especially if your posture might have caused muscle imbalances in the rotator cuff. It is quite easy to push too hard with the working arm, and so take it slowly and build up to increasing the stretch.

The scapula foam roll is an effective exercise for the shoulders and targets the muscles around the scapulae. It works the same as any other foam-rolling exercise by mobilising the soft tissues and allowing you to maintain pressure on the sore and knotted tissues. As mentioned in the equipment chapter, the hardness of the foam roller will dictate how painful the process will be. A softer material is best to start with; you can then graduate to a harder material as the body area becomes more resilient.

1. To foam roll the muscles around the scapulae, lie down with your upper back on the foam roller. Plant your feet and raise your hips into the air.
2. Hug yourself by wrapping your arms around yourself to stretch your back muscles. This makes them more accessible and easier to target.
3. Roll backwards and forwards slowly on the roller over the muscles of the scapulae for 10 seconds, and then rest.

EXERCISE 5.8: DEAD HANG

Target Area: Shoulders, chest, back
Sets: 3
Duration: Hold for 20 seconds
Rest: 30–45 seconds

LEVEL 2

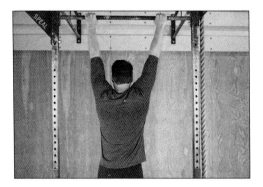

As the name suggests, this exercise involves hanging from a pull-up bar to activate the rotator cuff, and to stretch those muscles around the chest and back which pull on the shoulder. The dead hang puts a lot of demand on the hands, wrists, forearms and elbows, and so is a great overall conditioning exercise. Here, we are using it to target the shoulder where the distracting force at the joint develops the supportive function of the rotator cuff. The way the shoulders are positioned in this exercise is key to achieving maximum gains.

1. To perform the dead hang, grab a pull-up bar with both hands in an overhand grip position. Tuck your thumbs under the bar.
2. Now hang with straight arms, keeping the rest of your body relaxed. From here, pull your shoulders down so that they move away from your ears. Do not bend your elbows.
3. Hold this position for the required amount of time, and then rest.

Teaching Points

This version of the dead hang differs slightly from standard versions in that the aim here is to engage the shoulders and position the scapulae correctly. This is vital for developing this exercise into the scapula pull-up, which requires 'pulling' with the scapulae to improve their function and develop injury resistance. Concentrate on not bending the elbows; this will help in activating the correct muscles at the shoulder.

EXERCISE 5.9: SCAPULA PULL-UP

Target Area: Muscles around the scapulae
Sets: 3
Reps: 10
Rest: 30–45 seconds

LEVEL 2

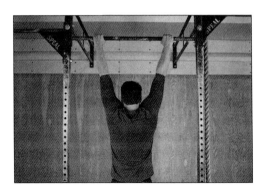

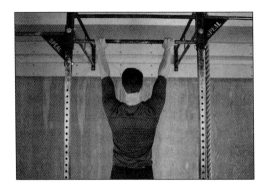

The scapula pull-up builds on the dead hang (Exercise 5.8), and when used correctly can effectively develop the supporting muscles of the shoulder. There are a number of stages to this exercise, allowing it to be adapted to a wide range of abilities. We will start with the normal version.

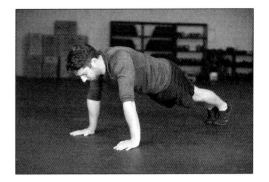

1. To perform the scapula pull-up, grab a pull-up bar with an overhand grip, hands positioned shoulder-width apart.
2. Hang with your elbows straight, allowing your shoulders to rise up to meet the ears. This is the starting position.
3. Using the muscles around the back and shoulders, pull your shoulders down so that they move away from your ears. You should reach a limit where they cannot move down any further. Hold this position for a few seconds.
4. Now allow your body to drop slowly so that you reach the starting position again. This counts as one repetition.

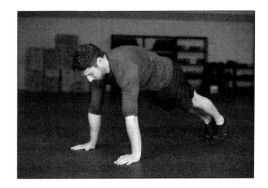

Teaching Points

If you have never done this type of exercise before, it is tempting to simply bend the elbows to complete the movement. However, this is more akin to a normal pull-up, and the intended target muscles will not be used. Make sure to keep your elbows relaxed and straight, and concentrate on pulling the shoulders down to get them as far away from your ears as possible.

EXERCISE 5.10: SCAPULA PUSH-UP

Primary Target Area: Rotator cuff muscles, muscles around the scapulae
Sets: 3
Reps: 10
Rest: 30–45 seconds   **LEVEL 1**

The scapula push-up is one of four scapula-specific strength exercises (the others being the dead hang, scapula dip and scapula pull-up). It is a great introductory exercise for developing the weight-bearing function of the shoulder. The exercise will increase your awareness of how to activate your shoulder muscles before progressing to more advanced body-weight exercises. The intention of the scapula exercises is not to develop the muscles worked in the push-up (such as the pectorals, triceps and deltoids), but rather to develop the muscles supporting the shoulder complex.

1. To perform the scapula push-up, assume a normal push-up position. Your hands should be flat on the floor, shoulder-width apart, and your legs should be straight, with your weight on your toes. Maintain a strong core with a neutral spine position.
2. From here, draw your shoulder blades apart so that your spine begins to rise.

Do not bend the elbows. This is the starting position.

3. Allow your spine to lower slowly so that your chest moves towards the floor and your shoulder blades move closer together. Do not bend the elbows, and keep your body as straight as possible.

4. Draw your shoulder blades apart again so that you return to the starting position. This counts as one repetition. Repeat for the required number of repetitions, and then rest.

Teaching Points

The hardest part about the scapula push-up (as with most scapula movements) is controlling the elbow joint. The elbows should remain straight throughout the exercise, in order to place the emphasis on the muscles of the shoulder complex. If you find this difficult at first, try to make the degree of movement smaller, concentrating on drawing the spine up and then down until the controlled ROM increases.

EXERCISE 5.11: BAR SHOULDER DISLOCATE

Primary Target Area: Shoulders
Sets: 1
Reps: 10   LEVEL 2

When the band shoulder dislocate (Key Exercise 5.4) becomes easy to perform, you can progress to the bar shoulder dislocate. This movement uses a straight, fixed bar instead of a band, which means that the hands have to stay the same width apart at all times. The bar that you use should be light and straight, with little weight to it. Broom handles or exercise class barbells (the light ones) are excellent for this.

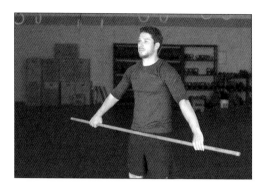

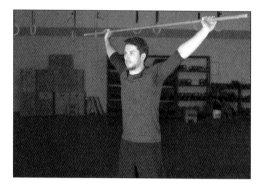

1. To perform the bar shoulder dislocate, grab a bar with both hands and hold it in front of your pelvis. Both elbows should be straight and your grip loose but strong. Begin with a wide grip.

2. Start to raise the bar up and over your head, keeping your elbows straight and your arms wide. If you cannot move the bar all the way over your head, move your hands further apart. It will take a little experimentation to find the right width.

3. If you are able, keep going until the bar reaches your lower back. At no point should you bend your elbows.

4. Reverse the movement until you reach the starting position. This counts as one repetition.

Teaching Points

The main sticking point with this exercise is using a grip that is too narrow. Begin with a wide grip and gradually narrow the grip as you progress. The aim is to get the hands as close together as possible while still executing the movement with perfect form.

EXERCISE 5.12: ONE-ARMED DEAD HANG

Target Area: Rotator cuff muscles, muscles around the scapulae
Sets: 5
Duration: as long as possible
Rest: 30–45 seconds   `LEVEL 3`

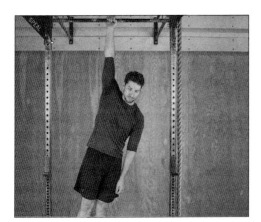

This exercise builds on the dead hang (Exercise 5.8), and is a progression to using just one arm. It will be more difficult, not just because of the extra body weight that your arm will be holding, but also because of the fact that your body will want to twist and rotate. There is also the issue of holding onto the bar with one hand; this will probably be difficult, even for those with good base strength, but practice is the only thing that will improve this strength.

1. To perform the one-armed dead hang, grab the pull-up bar with one arm in an overhand grip.
2. Now hang with a straight arm, keeping the rest of your body relaxed. You may have to bring your free arm across your chest to stop yourself from rotating or swinging. As before, pull your scapula down in the working arm.
3. Pull the shoulder of your working arm down, away from your ear. Do not bend the elbow.
4. Hold this position for as long as possible, and then rest. To ensure the development of both shoulders, you can repeat the exercise on the other arm.

Teaching Points

It is likely that many will find this exercise very difficult, but it is not impossible. The prerequisite is that you should spend a lot of time doing normal two-armed dead hangs before moving on to this version. Depending on your body weight and physical make-up, this movement will be more difficult or less difficult, but even a lighter person will struggle initially. Progress slowly and test yourself regularly, and you will soon be performing one-armed dead hangs.

EXERCISE 5.13: ONE-HANDED SCAPULA PULL-UP

Target Area: Rotator cuff muscles, muscles around the scapulae
Sets: 3
Reps: 5
Rest: 30–45 seconds   `LEVEL 3`

Building on the one-armed dead hang (Exercise 5.12), we arrive at the one-handed scapula pull-up. Here, the body is raised up and down, for a given number of repetitions, using the muscles of the shoulder and upper back to engage the scapula and strengthen the area.

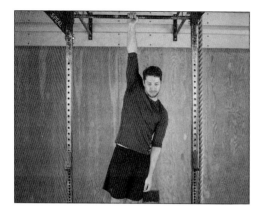

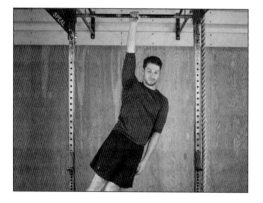

1. To perform the one-handed scapula pull-up, grab a pull-up bar with one hand in an overhand grip.
2. Hang with your elbow straight, allowing your shoulder to rise up to meet your ear. This is the starting position.
3. Using the muscles of the shoulder and back pull your shoulder down so that it moves away from your ear. You should reach a limit where you cannot pull yourself up any further. Hold this position for a second.
4. Allow your body to lower slowly so that you reach the starting position again. This counts as one repetition.

Teaching Points

In addition to the difficulty of this exercise, you may find it challenging to stop yourself from spinning when holding onto the bar with a single hand. To remedy this, you can hang a towel or piece of rope from the bar and hold this with your free hand. This will stop you from spinning, but you must make sure to only use the working arm to pull with.

You may also struggle to hold onto the bar for any length of time with only one hand. To rectify this simply spend time hanging from the bar, both with one hand and with two. Over time you will build enough strength to be able to perform this exercise.

■ Goal Exercises for the Shoulder

The exercises given in this chapter so far have been about building ROM, flexibility, stability and strength for injury prevention in the shoulder region and for making this region injury-proof. When performing those exercises, you will have noticed that they are working multiple areas of the body, giving you a fuller workout and a more functional level of conditioning. In this next part, we are going to examine some goal exercises that you should be aiming to perform as a test of both proper function and general strength and fitness. These exercises can be thought of as the 'standards' for each body zone, and are included here to promote your overall physical development.

GOAL EXERCISE 5.14: GERMAN HANG

Target Area: Shoulders
Sets: 3
Duration: Hold for 15 seconds
Rest: 30 seconds   **LEVEL 3**

This movement originates from gymnastics and is designed to strengthen and mobilise the

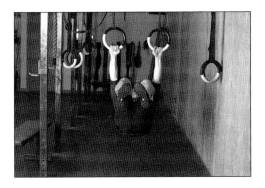

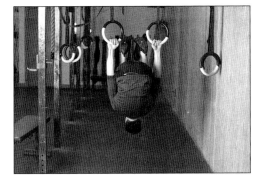

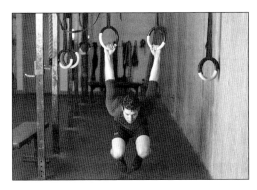

shoulder joint; it is great for those looking to injury-proof this area of the body. The German hang can be performed on a pull-up bar or with gymnastic rings. Rings are our preferred method, because pull-up bars are normally situated above head height, and so a fall can be dangerous. Gymnastic rings, on the other hand, can be lowered to waist height, making the movement safer and easier to learn.

1. To perform the German hang, grab the pull-up bar or gymnastic rings with an overhand grip.

2. Keeping your arms straight, tuck your knees into your chest. The closer you can get your knees to your chest the better, as this will make the subsequent rotation easier.

3. Now pull down as hard as you can, aiming to get your legs through the gap in your arms.

4. Keep rotating around until your legs are free of your arms. Next, let your legs straighten and relax so that they point at the ground. You should now be able to see the floor, and your arms should remain straight.

5. Hold this position for as long as you can, aiming for 15–20 seconds. When you get tired or reach the time limit, let go of the bar and land on your feet.

Teaching Points

One of the main sticking points of the German hang is the issue of going upside down. There is both a fear and a physical element to this. The fear element will disappear with time and confidence, but the physical element is different. If you are having trouble rotating all the way around, make sure that your legs are tucked tightly into your chest and that your knees are bent; this will keep your weight centred and rotation will be easier. Be aware that the German hang is a more difficult exercise and is included as a progression of your body-weight training.

GOAL EXERCISE 5.15: PUSH-UP

Target Area: Triceps, deltoids, pectorals
Sets: 3
Reps: 10–20
Rest: 30–45 seconds

LEVEL 1

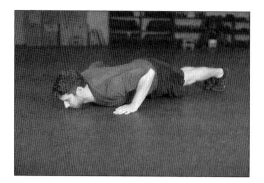

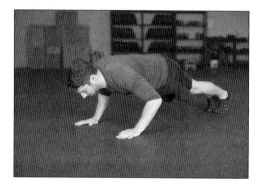

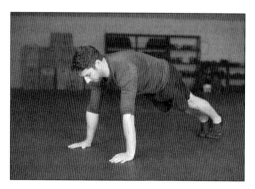

2. Balance on your toes so that a straight line can be drawn through the shoulders, hips and ankles. Maintain a strong core and a neutral spine position.

3. Bend the elbows and start to lower your chest towards the ground. Make sure that your hips do not sag or drop lower than your shoulders. Do not allow the head to protract forwards, and keep the neck neutral and relaxed.

4. Keep lowering until your chest touches the ground. Pause for a second, and then push back up again until your elbows straighten. This counts as one repetition.

Teaching Points

As with other exercises where the body weight is supported on the hands, making the push-up easier is achieved by placing the hands on a raised platform. The step described in the equipment chapter (Chapter 3) will be perfect for this. The rule here is that the higher the platform, the easier the movement; conversely, the lower the platform, the harder the movement. If you are struggling to perform the exercise, begin with the platform at waist height. As you get stronger, you will be able to gradually reduce the height of this platform until you are strong enough to perform the movement on the floor.

The push-up is very well known, and one of the most fundamental body-weight exercises that exists. It is used in the military, in exercise classes, by those who train at home and by anyone who is looking to build strength in their upper body. It is classed as a *pushing exercise*, in that the arms are moving away from the body.

1. To perform the push-up, place both hands flat on the ground, shoulder-width apart, and stretch your legs out behind you.

GOAL EXERCISE 5.16: TRICEPS DIP

Target Area: Triceps, deltoids, pectorals
Sets: 3
Reps: 5–10
Rest: 45–60 seconds

LEVEL 2

The triceps dip is the second pushing exercise in this part, but is more difficult than the push-up; the main reason is that the upper body is supporting the entire body weight.

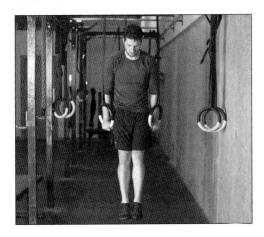

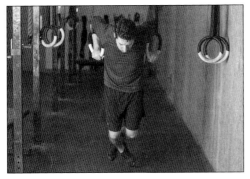

The dip has often been called the upper body equivalent of the squat, and for good reason. It will develop strength throughout the entire upper body, with the chest, triceps and shoulders doing a very large amount of work.

1. To perform the triceps dip, grab a set of dip bars with your palms facing inwards.
2. Push up until your arms are straight, or jump into the air and 'catch' yourself in the top position.
3. Push down and raise your torso so that your ears move away from your shoulders (as in Key Exercise 5.1 – scapula dip). This is the starting position.
4. From here, bend your elbows and start to lower your body towards the ground. Allow your shoulders to move forwards if necessary, and cross your feet and tuck them behind you if they will touch the ground.

5. Keep bending your elbows until you reach the limit of your ROM; this may be at the right-angle position. Pause for a second, and then push back up until you reach the starting position. This counts as one repetition.

Teaching Points

The dip is a difficult exercise for beginners, but there are ways to make it more manageable. One method is to work with the negative phase of the exercise, which is moving with gravity but controlling the rate of descent. Start at the top of the movement, and then lower yourself towards the ground as slowly as possible. Once you reach the limit of your ROM, drop off the bar. This will count as one repetition, and will be much more effective at building strength than doing the exercise with a reduced ROM. As you get stronger, you will be able to start pushing up from the bottom position.

GOAL EXERCISE 5.17: PULL-UP

Target Area: Biceps, latissimus dorsi
Sets: 3
Reps: 5–10
Rest: 30–45 seconds   LEVEL 2

The pull-up is the king of body-weight exercises, and is still used as a strength marker for many professions that rely on physical fitness, including the military and law enforcement. In the sports world the pull-up is the basis of much upper body training, from gymnasts to football and hockey players. It differs from the negative chin-up in the way the hands grab the bar: in a chin-up the hands are positioned in an underhand grip, which allows a slightly stronger pull. The pull-up,

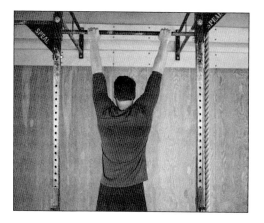

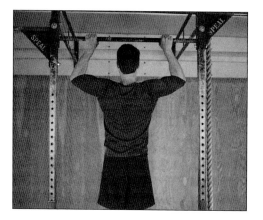

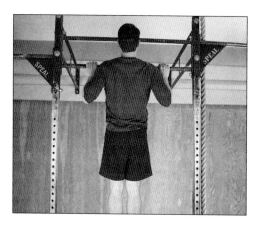

the pull-up is more difficult than the chin-up, but more beneficial in terms of upper body strength building.

1. To perform the pull-up, grab a pull-up bar in an overhand grip. Your hands should be slightly wider than shoulder width, or in whatever position feels the most natural and comfortable.
2. Hang with your legs straight, and allow your shoulders to rise up to meet your ears. This is the starting position.
3. From here, engage your scapula muscles (as in the scapula pull-up – Exercise 5.9), and pull your shoulders down so that they move away from your ears. Do not bend your elbows as you do this.
4. Start to pull with your arms and back. Your elbows will bend as you do this; allow them to flare out to the sides as far as comfort allows.
5. Keep pulling until your chin reaches over the bar, or your chest touches the bar. Pause for a second, and then return under control to the starting position.

Teaching Points

For many people, performing a perfect pull-up eludes them, even after they have been training for many years. There can be a number of reasons why this is the case. First, ensure that you start the pull-up movement with straight arms. Starting with bent arms makes the movement easier, but it does not help to develop strength throughout the whole ROM. The best method is to use the negative phase of the movement: this requires you to start at the top of the movement (with your chin over the bar), and finish at the bottom of the movement. To do this you will need to stand on a platform underneath the pull-up bar. Grab the bar with loose elbows, and then jump into the air. As you do this,

however, is performed with an overhand grip, which allows the hands to be positioned wider, opens up the chest and relies more on the strength of the upper back. As a result, pull hard and aim to get your chin over the bar. Once in the top position, slowly lower yourself down towards the ground under control. Once your arms become straight, drop off the bar. This counts as one repetition.

As you get stronger, you will be able to start pulling up from the bottom position, until you can perform the full movement properly.

6

The Elbow

Introduction to the Elbow

Together with the shoulder, the elbow works
to manipulate the position of the hand
relative to the world around us. Unlike the
shoulder, however, which allows a large
ROM in multiple directions, the elbow joint
is relatively straightforward. The elbow is
probably most noteworthy for its muscular
double-act – the biceps and triceps muscles.
It is also well known for its susceptibility to
injuries linked to sporting actions: the nature
of golfer's elbow and tennis elbow will be
reviewed later in this chapter.

> **KEY POINT** *The elbow works with the
> shoulder to position the hand relative to
> the world around us.*

Functional Anatomy of the Elbow

Passive Structures
Technically speaking, the elbow consists of
two joints: 1) a hinge joint, or the 'true' or
proper elbow joint, for flexion and extension
movements; and 2) a pivot joint, called the
superior (upper) radioulnar joint, for rotational
movements. As the name suggests, the second
joint is created by the joining of the two
long bones of the forearm – the radius and
the ulna. When you turn your palm up and
down it is this second elbow joint that allows
the forearm bones to rotate relative to one
another. The radius and the ulna, along with
the humerus, make up the bony anatomy of
the elbow, shown in Figure 6.1.

Like all the moveable joints discussed in this
book, the elbow joints are surrounded by

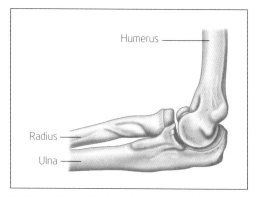

Humerus

Radius

Ulna

■ **Figure 6.1.** Basic anatomy of the right
elbow joint: medial view in 90-degree flexion.

a weak joint capsule to contain the lubricating joint fluid. The capsule is reinforced by strong ligaments, some of which might be strained as a result of repetitive throwing stress. This can give rise to a condition in adults that is similar to 'little-league' elbow in children, a condition more common where baseball pitching is a regular sporting movement.

Active Structures

There are, perhaps surprisingly, many muscles either crossing or acting on the elbow joint (Figure 6.2). There are 13 to be exact, but we will concern ourselves with only a few muscles or groups of muscles, specifically:

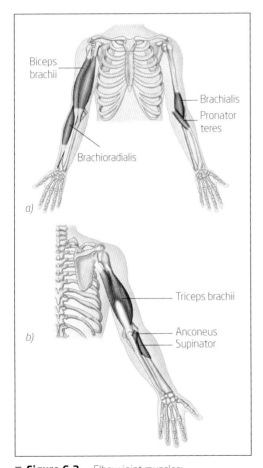

■ **Figure 6.2.** Elbow joint muscles:
(a) anterior view; (b) posterior view.

- Biceps
- Triceps
- Forearm flexors
- Forearm extensors

There are others not mentioned in the list above that contribute to turning the palm up or down, or that assist in flexion and extension of the elbow. The ones selected above have been singled out because they cross more than one joint, and so can be prone to strain injury. These muscles contract and shorten, pulling on their tendons and drawing the anchoring bones closer together. Of the muscles listed above, it is probably the two-headed biceps that has the most demands placed upon it. As we saw in Chapter 5 of this book, the upper tendon of the biceps can be injured as it crosses the shoulder. Then there is the bulk of muscle at the front of the arm that can be subject to tremendous strain. Finally, we have the tendon at the elbow, which flexes the joint and pulls on the radius bone to turn the palm upwards. These different functions have given rise to numerous variations of the biceps curl, as seen in your local gym.

The antagonist of the biceps muscle is the triceps muscle; this three-headed beast pulls on the elbow in the opposite direction, to cause extension. In addition to the biceps and triceps, there are opposing groups of muscles acting from below the elbow.

The muscle groups known as the *forearm flexors and extensors*, as shown in Figure 6.3, originate from the bony bumps on the outer and inner parts of your elbow. These muscles cross both the elbow and the wrist, and so are under dual strain, making them more susceptible to injury. Repeated movements, such as gripping or flicking the wrist, can cause the familiar tennis and golfer's elbow conditions, which are discussed in detail later.

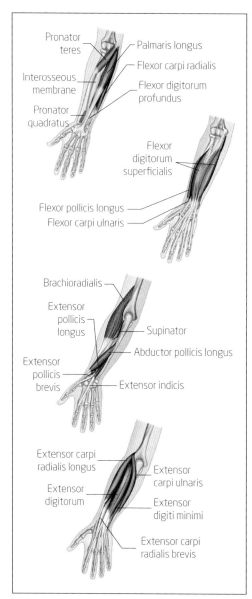

■ **Figure 6.3.** The forearm flexor and extensor muscle groups.

In normal daily movements, the muscles outlined above act on the joints to pull the upper limbs freely through the air (by this we mean that generally the hand is not fixed – think of a biceps curl exercise or handwriting). When you perform body-weight exercises, however, like those described in Chapters 5, 6 and 7 of this book, something different occurs – the hand is generally fixed. This means that the body moves relative to the hand (think of a push-up or pull-up). These movements now create a weight-bearing stability demand on the wrist, elbow and shoulder, and develop the stabilising and control ability of the muscles involved. When the load is progressively increased, these exercises also develop amazing strength, as can be seen in more advanced calisthenics exercises.

> **KEY POINT** *Whether it is our childhood physical development, or a link to our evolutionary ancestors, humans are no strangers to using the upper limbs for pushing, pulling, hanging, swinging and crawling.*

At first glance, the previous paragraph may seem to contradict the whole ethos of this book: we have so far extolled the benefits of 'functional' exercise and activity. So why on earth would bearing weight through the arms be regarded as functional? If you cast your mind back as far as your early physical development, you may recall that pushing, pulling, hanging, swinging and crawling were all common in your movement repertoire. And it was not too far back in our evolutionary history that the precursors to our species walked intermittently on their upper limbs and climbed trees regularly. While we are not suggesting that we all revert to the behaviour of our evolutionary ancestors, perhaps the 'chimp' or child in all of us needs exercising from time to time!

Before we explore some body-weight exercises to load the upper limbs, let's explore some common elbow problems that would benefit from bulletproofing exercise.

■ Common Elbow Dysfunction

Tennis Elbow

Tennis elbow is the most common elbow complaint and can also be one of the most difficult to manage and resolve (Figure 6.4). It is often regarded as a chronic problem, meaning that it has persisted for more than six weeks; however, it is usually at least three months before some sort of action is taken. Our advice is to start management of this condition early, and this is likely to involve loading exercises. If you are unsure as to how to proceed, we recommend that you seek the advice of a qualified health or medical professional.

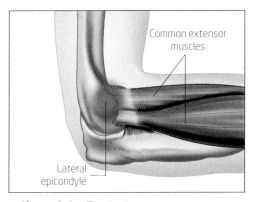

Common extensor muscles

Lateral epicondyle

■ **Figure 6.4.**   Tennis elbow.

The pain of tennis elbow is usually felt on the outer aspect of the elbow, on or just below the bony bump; this is the site of a common tendon attachment for many of the muscles of the forearm. As outlined above, it is the extensor muscle group that attaches on the outer side of the elbow, and so movements involving heavy or repeated gripping can strain this region. Try gripping without cocking your wrist back and you will begin to appreciate the role of the extensor muscle group muscles and their common tendon. If you add more extension stress at the wrist, such as a tennis backhand stroke or the use

of a plastering trowel, you may be on your way to developing tennis elbow.

The peak age of onset of tennis elbow is between 35 and 54, and the majority of cases are caused by work-related activities. Rather than being an inflammatory problem, tennis elbow is commonly regarded as a *tendinopathy*, suggesting some degree of tendon breakdown or disruption of its fibres. Management of this problem should therefore involve identifying and modifying aggravating movements; where this is not possible, we recommended developing physical resilience and improved function around the elbow with loaded exercise. Try body-weight Key Exercise 6.1 for starters.

KEY EXERCISE 6.1: INVERTED-WRIST WALL PUSH-UP

Target Area: Elbows, forearms, chest, shoulders
Sets: 3
Reps: 5–20, depending on strength
Rest: 30 seconds   **LEVEL 2**

As we have seen, the wrist extensor muscle group operates at both the wrist and the elbow. With the inverted-wrist wall push-up, we can effectively target the muscle during both functions and develop a gradual load on the common tendon. If you have tennis elbow, you may find discomfort when performing this exercise, and so build up slowly. If you are prone to tennis elbow but are currently pain-free, this exercise will improve the chances of staying pain-free.

1. Stand in front of a solid wall, far enough back so that you can lean into the wall with outstretched arms. Now the tricky

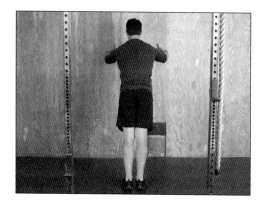

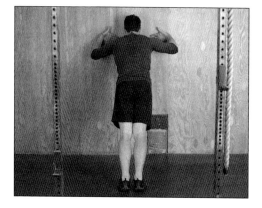

the depth of the push-up. To make it harder, the same principles apply. Focus on the wrist and forearm involvement rather than aiming to work the chest. If you do suffer from tennis elbow, you will quite likely need to continue with this exercise for a few months before your body makes the necessary adaptations. Stick with it!

Also recommended: Key Exercise 7.2 (forearm and wrist stretch 2), Key Exercise 7.4 (inverted-wrist push-up support), Exercise 7.8 (kneeling inverted-wrist push-up).

bit – lean against the wall with the backs of your hands (inverted). Try this with your fingers either pointing downwards or slightly in towards the other hand. Adjust your lean to make the pressure on the wrist and hands more comfortable.

2. Slowly lower your chest towards the wall, allowing your elbows to flex (bend). Take this movement as far as your strength allows. Pause for a second at the end of the movement, and then slowly return to the starting position. Throughout, ensure that you are engaging the wrist extensor muscles to control the back of your hand against the wall.

3. Repeat.

Teaching Points

The degree of difficulty of this exercise can easily be changed by altering your standing position relative to the wall and by reducing

Golfer's Elbow

Golfer's elbow (Figure 6.5) has a very similar cause, process and presentation to tennis elbow as described previously. It is less common than tennis elbow, but when it does occur it can be painful and affect function. With golfer's elbow, the pain will be experienced at the bony bump on the inner part of the elbow. It may be tender to touch but will most often be aggravated by the use of the wrist or elbow. When moving from a resting position, the elbow may feel stiff and painful.

It is the wrist flexor muscle group that becomes problematic in golfer's elbow; as with

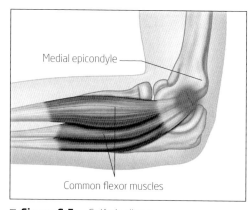

Medial epicondyle

Common flexor muscles

■ **Figure 6.5.** Golfer's elbow.

tennis elbow, it is the attachment of the common tendon that starts to be troublesome. Unaccustomed use of the flexor muscle group causes breakdown and disruption of the flexor tendon. Once again, we advise a thorough assessment of aggravating movements, with subsequent modification of activity. This should be supplemented with a prolonged period of loading to the tendon and muscles, allowing time for the structures to adapt to the progressive stress. If you are unsure, seek the advice of a health or medical professional. Once you feel able to begin loaded exercise, try the body-weight winner Key Exercise 6.2.

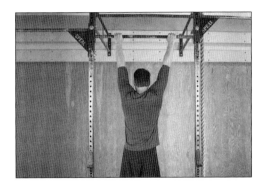

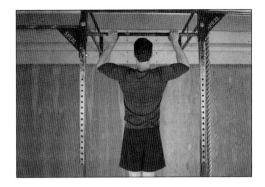

KEY EXERCISE 6.2: PULL-UP/ STATIC HANG

Target Area: Elbows, forearms, back muscles
Sets: 3
Reps: 1–20, depending on strength
Rest: 45–60 seconds   **LEVEL 2**

The pull-up is a foundation of body-weight exercise, and can be a secret weapon against golfer's elbow. By using an overhand grip of the bar, you automatically engage the wrist flexor muscle group. When pulling on the bar to create the pull-up, the elbow must bend, and it is here that the wrist flexor muscles are subjected to their second loading. The rest of the effort comes from the large muscles of the back. If you cannot complete a pull-up, simply try the initiating movement, or the 'static hold' outlined in the teaching points.

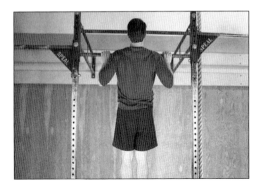

1. Grasp a pull-up bar with an overhand grip. Your hands should be about shoulder-width apart or slightly wider.
2. Hang with the elbows straight – this is a dead hang. It is important for protecting against golfer's elbow that the elbow is able to straighten at the lowest part of the pull-up. It makes the pull-up more difficult, but do not cheat on this.
3. Before you start the pull, shrug your shoulders down first, as demonstrated in Exercise 5.9. Now pull yourself towards the bar, keeping your hips reasonably straight. If able, reach your chest or chin to the bar. Do not be tempted to swing or lift your knees forwards.

4. From the top position, lower yourself down to the starting position, until your elbows straighten again. This is one repetition. Repeat as able.

Teaching Points

If you struggle to perform the pull-up, try a static hold. After grabbing the bar with an overhand grip, assume the pull-up position you wish to hold. If this is the top position, use a step or box to get up to the bar. You can also lower yourself slowly from this position; this is an *eccentric* loading exercise.

Also recommended: Key Exercise 7.1 (forearm and wrist stretch 1), Exercise 7.3 (push-up support), Exercise 7.7 (false-grip hang).

Bursitis

As mentioned in Chapter 5 (shoulder) and Chapter 9 (knee), a *bursa* (pl. *bursae*) is a fluid-filled sac, which can become swollen or inflamed when subjected to repeated friction or pressure. Bursitis (the swelling of a bursa) can also happen as a result of a direct trauma, but such an injury is not the focus of this book; in this instance, you are directed to seek information on managing acute injuries.

The bursa in question at the elbow is called the *olecranon bursa*; it is so called because it sits alongside the bony olecranon bump at the back of the elbow. This bursa reduces friction between the olecranon bump and the triceps tendon as it pulls to straighten the elbow. Pressure may occur with prolonged or repeated leaning on the back of the elbow (*student's elbow*).

Elbow bursitis (Figure 6.6) may also be the result of repeated straightening of the elbow against load, especially where the pull of the triceps is focused at the elbow because the arm is fixed by the side. One such cause is the gym-based triceps extension exercise: here, the action of the triceps at the shoulder is immobilised and the muscle pull is entirely directed at the elbow through a limited ROM. Once the acute phase of olecranon bursitis has settled, replace your resisted triceps extensions with a body-weight exercise, such as Key Exercise 6.3.

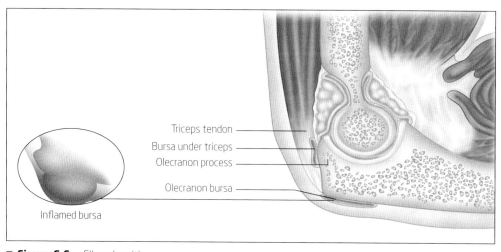

Triceps tendon
Bursa under triceps
Olecranon process
Olecranon bursa
Inflamed bursa

■ **Figure 6.6.** Elbow bursitis.

KEY EXERCISE 6.3: LEDGE DIP

Target Area: Elbows, shoulders
Sets: 3
Reps: 10
Rest: 45–60 seconds

LEVEL 1

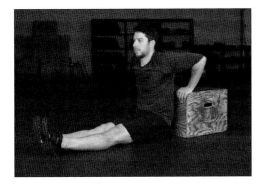

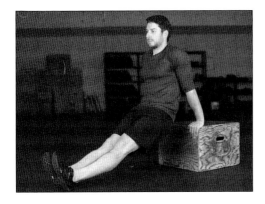

The ledge dip is a precursor to the fully-fledged triceps dip, but does not require any specialised equipment to perform. The ledge dip is also easier than the triceps dip, but it will still increase strength and resilience around the elbow joint, without overstressing the olecranon bursa. It will also develop some mobility and flexibility in the shoulder joint as well.

1. To perform the ledge dip, place your hands behind you on an exercise box, bench, step or raised platform, with your fingers facing forwards. You can even use a windowsill or a kitchen worktop, as long as it is stable and safe. Your hands should be shoulder-width apart. Try a height of around 30–45cm or so for the platform.
2. Stretch your legs out and straighten your knees, balancing on your heels. Keep your back close to your hands.
3. Now bend your elbows and start to descend, until your elbows are bent at a 90-degree angle if possible. You may be limited here by your shoulder flexibility; if this is the case, just descend as far as your mobility allows.
4. Pause for a second, and then push up to return to the starting position. This counts as one repetition. Repeat.

Teaching Points

You may struggle to perform the ledge dip as described, mainly because of a lack of strength or mobility at either the shoulder or the elbow. This is the beauty of body-weight exercise, in that it simultaneously strengthens and mobilises multiple joints; this does, however, make the movements more challenging, but also more rewarding! To reduce the intensity of the movement, you can bend the knees and bring the feet in towards the hands. As you progress, you can straighten the legs out gradually and move on to the full version.

Biceps Tendon Problems

Pain with resisted elbow flexion (bending) or when turning the palm up may be due to a strain of the fleshy bulk of the biceps muscle or of the biceps tendon at its attachment on the radius bone. If the problem came on suddenly with heavy lifting, you may have torn some of the muscle or tendon fibres, or even ruptured the biceps tendon (Figure 6.7); in such cases, we recommend that you get

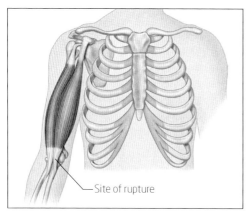

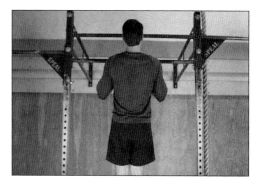

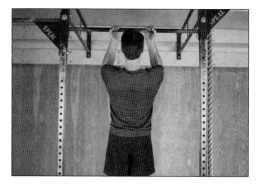

■ Figure 6.7. Biceps tendon rupture.

assessed by a health or medical professional. Once you have been cleared to start rehabilitation exercises, you can gradually build up your body-weight exercise routine. Even if you do not currently have an injury of the biceps, but want to increase your physical resilience here, then Key Exercise 6.4 is a great starting point.

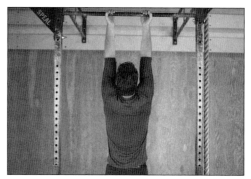

KEY EXERCISE 6.4: NEGATIVE CHIN-UP

Target Area: Elbows, shoulders, forearms
Sets: 3
Reps: 3–10
Rest: 45 seconds   **LEVEL 3**

One movement that is great for developing strength in and around the elbow joint is the negative chin-up. The negative phase of an exercise (also known as the *eccentric phase*) is moving with gravity, but without letting gravity dictate the pace. A negative chin-up therefore starts with your chin over the bar and finishes in a dead hang.

1. To perform the negative chin-up, stand on a raised box or platform underneath

a pull-up bar. The box should be high enough to allow you to grab the pull-up bar with bent elbows.

2. Grasp the bar with an underhand grip, hands slightly narrower than your shoulders.

3. Bend your knees and jump as high as you can, pulling with your arms so that you finish with your chin over the bar.

4. Hold this position for a second and make sure you are comfortable. Then lower

yourself down to the ground, using your biceps and back muscles to control the movement. Throughout the entire movement, make sure that your shoulder blades are drawn down, engaging the scapula muscles (see Chapter 5).

5. Keep lowering until your elbows are completely straight. This counts as one repetition. Repeat for the desired number of repetitions then rest.

Teaching Points

The negative chin-up will impart great strength and reduce the risk of injury around the elbow, precisely because of the amount of control that must be used to perform the exercise. It can be very stressful on the ligaments and tendons of the elbow, so maintain control of the movement. The negative chin-up uses eccentric loading, which is thought to quickly increase tendon and muscle strength.

Also recommended: Key Exercise 5.3 (chest stretch).

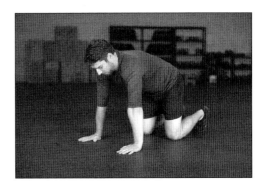

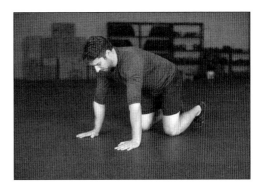

■ Body-weight Exercises for Improved Elbow Function

EXERCISE 6.5: ARM ROTATION

Target Area: Forearm/elbow muscles
Sets: 3
Reps: 10
Rest: 20 seconds   **LEVEL 1**

The arm rotation is a dynamic progression of the forearm and wrist stretch 1 (Key Exercise 7.1), and develops loading flexibility in the wrist flexor muscles. It also develops loading at the shoulder.

1. Crouch down on all fours, with your hands flat on the ground, shoulder-width apart.
2. From here, begin to rotate both of your arms inwards, while keeping your palms flat on the ground. This will require some practice, as it can be difficult to get the right muscles to activate.
3. Rotate your arms as far inwards as possible. You may feel the strain on the inner elbow. Hold at this point, and then reverse the movement, rotating the arms outwards (so that the inside of your elbow points forwards)
4. When you have returned to the start position, you have completed one repetition. Repeat.

Teaching Points

You may struggle to 'switch on' the right muscles and perform the movement correctly. Most of the activity comes from the shoulder, but we want you to focus on keeping the elbow straight and take up the strain in the forearm muscles that cross the elbow. Do not over-strain the shoulders with this exercise. Start with a small ROM at first, and the additional mobility will come with practice.

EXERCISE 6.6: FORKLIFT

Target Area: Elbows
Sets: 3
Reps: 5–10, as you are able
Rest: 30–45 seconds   **LEVEL 3**

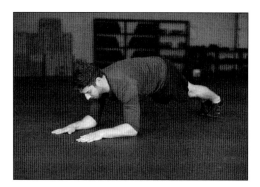

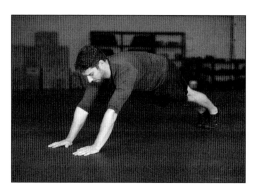

The forklift is a very unusual exercise that targets the outside of the elbow in an extremely effective manner. It is designed to eliminate the chest and shoulder muscles as much as possible during the pushing movement, and is therefore a lot more difficult than a normal push-up.

1. To perform the forklift, assume a push-up position. Your toes should be in contact with the ground, and your shoulders, hips and knees should form a straight line.
2. Now tuck your elbows into your sides, keeping them pointing towards the rear at all times. Start to bend your elbows and lower yourself towards the floor.
3. Keep moving towards the floor, until your forearms are flat against the ground. Make sure that your elbows point towards the rear. Once your forearms make contact with the ground, pause for a second.
4. From here, push back up to the start again, using mainly the triceps muscles. It is fine if the shoulders and chest do become involved, but try to limit their recruitment.

Teaching Points

This is a tough exercise and has been included here for those wishing to progress towards a complete calisthenics program. To make the forklift easier, you can move the hands further forward of the shoulders, as if in a Superman position; this allows the shoulders to help out more with the exercise. If it is still too difficult, you can adopt a kneeling position, as if you were doing a kneeling push-up; although this will be much easier than the normal version, it will still allow you to build strength and to progress.

EXERCISE 6.7: PLANCHE LEAN

Target Area: Elbows, shoulders
Sets: 3
Duration: Hold for 10 seconds
Rest: 30–45 seconds   **LEVEL 3**

As we have seen in this chapter, sports injuries in the elbow area can be so common that they even have sport-specific names

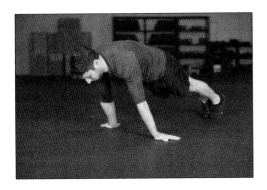

more advanced movements, such as the planche, handstand and exercises performed on the still rings. Start by only moving the shoulders a short way past the hands, and then gradually increase the distance as you get stronger.

■ Goal Exercises for the Elbow

Goal exercises are usually those that work multiple joints and muscles, but we have included some here that will give the elbow a good workout. As in the other chapters of this book, goal exercises can provide a benchmark test of your current abilities; however, the following exercises can also be used in a routine to develop overall bulletproof strength.

attributed to them: *tennis elbow*, *golfer's elbow* and so on. The planche lean builds additional strength and resilience in the elbow muscles and tendons by requiring the body to apply force with a straight arm. It is not for the faint-hearted!

1. To perform the planche lean, assume a normal push-up position.
2. Point your fingers backwards at an angle of approximately 45 degrees; this will then make the inside of your elbow point forwards. Make sure that your shoulders are directly over your hands.
3. From here, lean forwards or walk your toes forwards so that your shoulders move past your hands. You should feel pressure on your biceps, forearms and elbow joints.
4. Squeeze your shoulders together and push your spine towards the ceiling. Strive to keep your elbows straight, and 'pull' through the floor to maintain the hold.
5. Aim for a hold of 10 seconds, and then rest. Repeat.

Teaching Points

The planche lean will no doubt be difficult on your first few attempts, but this is expected, since we have included this exercise for those wanting to progress their physical resilience and body-weight strength. Gymnasts use this move in order to build up strength around the elbow joint to prepare them for

GOAL EXERCISE 6.8: ARCHER PUSH-UP

Target Area: Elbows, shoulders
Sets: 3
Reps: 5–20 each side
Rest: 45–60 seconds   **LEVEL 3**

A superb goal exercise for the elbow joint is the archer push-up. This is a little harder than a normal push-up, but the ROM can be adjusted quite dramatically, making it suitable for a wide range of abilities. It can also be performed on the knees, making it easier still.

1. To perform the archer push-up, assume the normal push-up position, but with the working hand positioned at 90 degrees, fingers pointing out to the sides. The hands should be slightly wider than normal.

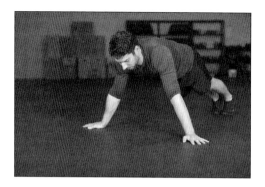

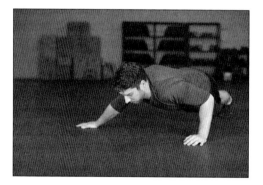

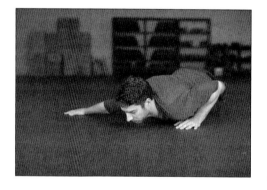

2. Bend your opposite arm and start to lower your chest to the floor. As you do this, move your upper body over to the side with the bent shoulder. Keep the opposite arm straight.

3. Keep descending towards the ground until your chest touches the floor. At this point, the opposite arm should be completely bent, and the working arm should be very close to the ground, but still straight.

4. From here, push up hard with the bent arm and 'pull' through the floor with the working arm. This will place the demand squarely on the elbow joint of the straight arm.

5. Keep rising until you reach the starting position. This counts as one repetition. Repeat the movement on the opposite side if you need more break between repetitions!

Teaching Points

The archer push-up can be made easier by reducing the ROM; in other words, you do not descend as far on each repetition, and so the working arm will not straighten completely. The exercise as detailed above can also be performed from a kneeling push-up position.

Also recommended: Goal Exercise 5.16 (triceps dip)

7

The Wrist

Introduction to the Wrist

The ability to manipulate the world around us is a major characteristic of humans that sets us apart from the rest of the animal kingdom. It is the wrist joint that couples the dexterous hand with the long levers of the arm. Not only does the wrist play a crucial role in dexterity but it also facilitates phenomenal grip strength through the passage of long tendons to the hand from the more powerful muscles of the forearm. For this reason, many of the exercises in this chapter are intimately linked to the exercises described for the elbow in Chapter 6.

With body-weight exercises, the relationship between the hand and the arm is often reversed, placing a different emphasis on the wrist joint. The hand normally moves freely on a fixed forearm, whereas in many body-weight exercises it is the hand that is fixed so that the arms, or even the entire body, can move; for example, think about the push-up exercise. Accordingly, this chapter will place great emphasis on the stability function of the upper limbs, and will demonstrate strengthening and stretching around the wrist through weight-bearing movements.

KEY POINT *With body-weight exercise, the wrist functions under load and reverses the relationship between the hand and arm by fixing the hand to create movement of the arm/body.*

Functional Anatomy of the Wrist

Passive Structures

The wrist and hand have many components that, for the most part, function together seamlessly. There are numerous small bones in the hand, and the two long bones of the forearm. The relationship of these passive structures can be seen in Figure 7.1.

As the radius and ulna bones run down towards the wrist joint, you will notice that it is the radius that provides the surface for the first row of carpal bones with which to articulate: this is the wrist joint. Figure 7.1 also shows the scaphoid bone on the inner row of the carpal bones; it is this bone that is commonly injured following a fall onto an outstretched hand. Bridging some of the gap between the lower end of the long ulna bone

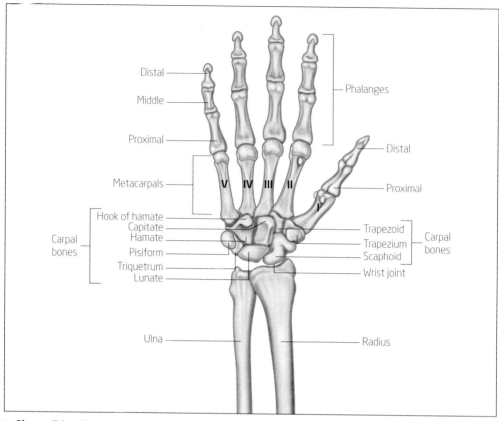

■ **Figure 7.1.** The bones of the wrist and hand.

with the row of carpal bones is a fibrous disc made of cartilage; this structure can also be injured in a fall, or may be subject to wear and tear as the body ages. As with all the joints reviewed in this book, the wrist and hand are bound, supported and restricted by ligaments; there are lots of ligaments between the numerous bones in this region!

The various movements provided by the wrist include some side-to-side 'deviations', while most movement involves flexion (palm to forearm) and extension (back of hand to forearm). Movements to turn the palm of the hand up and down (supination and pronation) do not derive from the wrist, but instead come from the rotation of the radius about the ulna (this action is considered

further in Chapter 6 for the elbow). Of course, none of these movements would be possible if it was not for the muscles and tendons pulling on the bones. Before we move on to these all-important active structures, it is worth considering one more passive structure that is unique to the wrist – the carpal tunnel.

The *carpal tunnel*, as depicted in Figure 7.2, is a strong fibrous band running across the wrist joint, below the palm of the hand. As this band runs over the carpal bones, it creates a tunnel for several structures to run under; these include the tendons we are about to discuss, but also some blood vessels and a nerve. You may already begin to visualise how irritation of the nerve in this tunnel could cause symptoms in the hand. We will

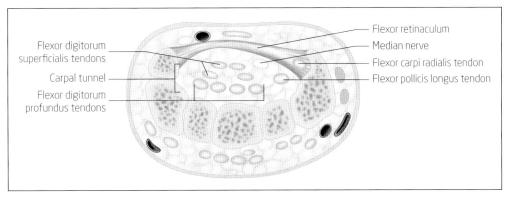

■ **Figure 7.2.** Here is a cross-section of the carpal tunnel, clearly showing the interrelationship between the muscles and associated structures.

examine this further when we get to the section on the common problems affecting the wrist and hand.

Active Structures

The hand houses numerous small muscles that create dexterity by manipulating the thumb and fingers. The muscles mostly responsible for these finer movements start and finish in the hand, and therefore do not cross the wrist joint. The muscles responsible for generating much of the power at the wrist and hand actually begin at the elbow and forearm. Try it for yourself – wiggle your fingers up and down as if typing, and watch what happens to the fleshy part of your forearm just below your outer elbow. The exercises outlined in this chapter may therefore contribute to improved function and reduced pain at the elbow as well as the wrist.

> **KEY POINT** *The muscles responsible for generating much of the power at the wrist and hand actually begin at the elbow and forearm.*

The larger muscles of the forearm taper into long, thin tendons that cross the wrist on its front and back surfaces. Some of the tendons heading over the back of the wrist and hand actually cross over each other and provide a potential point of friction, as will be explained later in this chapter. On the palm side of the wrist, some of the long tendons will run through the carpal tunnel and may therefore contribute to carpal tunnel syndrome. Figure 7.3 shows some of the muscles on the front and back of the forearm and wrist.

As with all the chapters in this book, you will see that the anatomy produces some very long and complicated names for the various structures. The good news is that we will not need to concentrate on individual named muscles, but instead we will develop complete functional strength and resilience in the forearm, wrist and hand.

■ Common Wrist Dysfunction

Injuries to the wrist and hand can be diverse, from a traumatic fall onto an outstretched hand to an overuse disorder from repetitive strain. Wherever possible, we advocate that prevention of injury is better than cure, but we appreciate that accidental falls or work-related stresses cannot always be avoided.

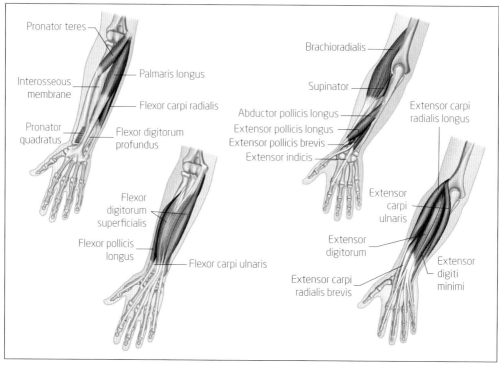

■ Figure 7.3. Muscles acting on the wrist.

By developing and maintaining a good level of physical resilience in the upper limbs and shoulders, however, it may be possible to limit the effects of such types of trauma should they occur. We will next explore some common wrist-related problems, and identify some suitable body-weight exercises to rehabilitate or injury-proof this vulnerable body area.

Wrist and Hand Joint Problems

Stiffness of the wrist, accompanied by a general restriction of movement, often indicates some sort of arthritis. Osteoarthritis, the wear-and-tear type of arthritis, tends to be less common in the wrist. If you have stiffness in both wrists, we recommend a review by a qualified health or medical professional before starting any new exercise programs. Osteoarthritis tends to more commonly affect the thumb joint and the finger-end joints. If you do not have the ROM in these joints to comfortably bear

weight through the hands, please modify all the exercises included here to allow progressive ROM and weight bearing. Begin with the basic stretch in Key Exercise 7.1 to increase the ability of the wrist to extend backwards under load, but please progress slowly!

KEY EXERCISE 7.1: FOREARM AND WRIST STRETCH 1

Target Area: Wrists, forearms
Sets: 3
Duration: 20 seconds
Rest: 20 seconds   **LEVEL 1**

A major part of injury prevention is making sure that the body is not limited in terms of the ROM that it can achieve. Stretching and mobilising the joints and surrounding soft tissues is therefore very important. The

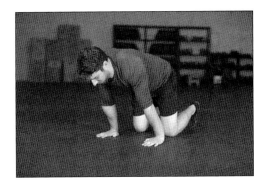

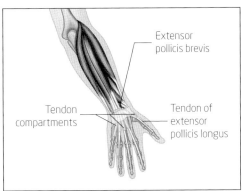

■ **Figure 7.4.** Wrist tenosynovitis.

forearm and wrist stretch 1, as we have called it, focuses on the wrist flexor muscles and takes the joint into an extended functional position that is crucial for maintaining grip strength. This is the reason why we have included this fundamental movement as a key exercise.

1. To perform forearm stretch 1, crouch down on your knees and place your palms flat on the floor, fingers facing forwards.
2. Keeping the heels of your palms pressed into the ground, lean forwards slowly until you feel the stretch on the underside of your forearms.
3. Hold this position for 20 seconds, and then relax. Repeat.

Teaching Points

Many people are surprised at how much this exercise stretches the muscles of the forearm. You may even feel it pull at the elbow if you have had symptoms suggestive of golfer's elbow (see Chapter 6). If you find that you cannot move forwards very far, keep increasing the stretch little by little during the weeks and months that you train. You will soon see an increase in flexibility and mobility in this area.

Tenosynovitis

Overuse is the most likely culprit of this common type of wrist problem, which involves irritation of the tendon and its surrounding sheath (Figure 7.4). The sheath in which the tendon runs can become thickened, and you may feel a soft-tissue creaking sensation as you work the muscles of the wrist and forearm. Most commonly, this sensation occurs on the radius bone side of the lower forearm as it runs towards the base of the thumb, but may also occur on the ulna side of the wrist as the tendon runs to the base of the little finger. Occasionally, a similar problem can occur higher up in the forearm, about three finger widths above the wrist: this is referred to as *oarsman's wrist*, because of its initial identification in rowers.

Most often, these conditions are part of a work- or leisure-related repetitive strain injury, and so identifying and addressing the cause of the problem should be your first priority. It may be that the 'problem' cannot be addressed, and that you simply have to carry out that work duty or hit that backhand stroke in tennis. In this instance, it may be a case of hardening your body to the stresses imposed on it. By making yourself more physically resilient to stress and strain, you will be well on your way to achieving that bulletproof body. Key exercise 7.2 is a great place to start for a tenosynovitis-type problem.

KEY EXERCISE 7.2: FOREARM AND WRIST STRETCH 2

Target Area: Wrists, forearms
Sets: 3
Duration: 20 seconds
Rest: 20 seconds   **LEVEL 1**

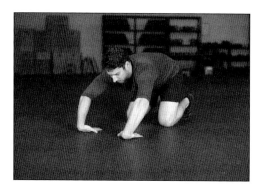

Since muscles work in opposing pairs, we must consider both groups when stretching. Forearm and Wrist Stretch 2 targets the wrist extensors, or the muscles that open the hand and wrist. This stretch is important with regard to some of the more difficult exercises in this chapter, like the inverted-wrist push-up, which requires considerable wrist and forearm flexibility.

1. To perform the forearm and wrist stretch 2, crouch down on your knees and place the backs of your hands flat on the floor, fingers facing backwards. Aim to keep your elbows as straight as possible. This may feel slightly awkward at first, but stick with it.
2. Keeping the backs of your hands pressed into the ground, lean backwards slowly until you feel the stretch on the top side of your forearms.

3. Hold this position for 20 seconds. Relax and repeat.

Teaching Points

This stretch is felt more strongly than Key Exercise 7.1 by most people, because the forearm extensors tend to be tighter than the flexors. Go slowly at first and do not overstretch these muscles. Build up the level of stretch over time in a gradual manner.

Wrist Tendon Problems

The site at which a tendon anchors to bone can often be a source of pain and dysfunction. There may be inflammation here, but more often than not it tends to be some degree of degenerative change in the tendon. There is good evidence to support the use of tendon loading as an effective treatment, but this may take weeks or months to work; therefore, stick with these body-weight exercises as long as they do not increase your pain. In such instances, we recommend assessment by a suitably qualified health or medical professional.

The site of dysfunction may be local to the site of tendon attachment, and commonly this will be on either side at the back of the wrist, or on the palm side of the wrist in line with the little finger. Tendon problems, or *tendinopathies*, may be due to repetitive overuse, and so it is worth taking time to see where you can modify your activities. When this is not possible, we recommend developing physical resilience in these tendons. Key Exercise 7.3 is offered as a starting point. If the tendinopathy is affecting the back of your wrist, try Key Exercise 7.4.

KEY EXERCISE 7.3: PUSH-UP SUPPORT

Target Area: Wrists, forearms
Sets: 3
Duration: 20 seconds
Rest: 20 seconds

LEVEL 1

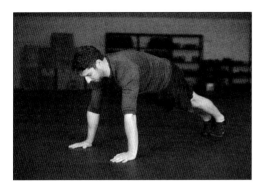

The most straightforward way to build strength in the hands and wrists is to simply hold a static push-up position. This is very similar in body position to the plank (Key Exercise 11.5), and so will also condition your spine and trunk; however, instead of supporting your body weight on the forearms, the hands take the majority of the load. A demand is placed on the muscles and connective tissues of the wrists and forearms, which in turn builds strength and flexibility in them.

1. To perform the push-up support, kneel on the ground and place your hands in front of you. Your hands should be shoulder-width apart, with the fingers splayed to aid balance.
2. Move your legs backwards and balance on your toes so that a straight line can be drawn through the shoulders, hips and ankles.
3. Hold this position for the required time, and then rest. Repeat.

Teaching Points

If you find this exercise too difficult, it can be made easier by placing the hands on a raised platform. Raising the hands will move more of your body weight onto the lower body. As you progress, you can reduce the height of the platform until you can perform the movement on level ground.

KEY EXERCISE 7.4: INVERTED-WRIST PUSH-UP SUPPORT

Target Area: Wrists, forearms
Sets: 3
Duration: 10–20 seconds, if possible.
Rest: 30–45 seconds
Rest: 20 seconds

LEVEL 3

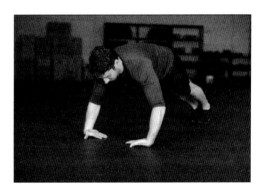

Note: *Not recommended when symptoms of carpal tunnel syndrome are present.*

The inverted-wrist push-up support is another great bulletproof movement that is a little unorthodox. Unless you have performed this type of movement before, you are likely to find it very difficult. With gradual practice, this exercise will help to strengthen the wrists in a stressed position, building resilience and helping to fend off injury.

1. To perform the inverted-wrist push-up support, crouch down and place the backs of your hands on the floor, fingers pointing inwards.
2. Stretch your legs out behind you and balance on your toes, as if you are in the top position of a push-up.
3. It is unlikely that you will be able to straighten your elbows, but do not worry about this: it is simply a consequence of anatomy.
4. Hold this position for as long as possible. Rest and repeat.

Teaching Points

It is quite normal not to be able to hold this position for very long; if this applies to you, support yourself for as long as you can and then drop your knees down to the floor. Keep doing this, supporting yourself and then recovering, and over time your strength and ability will increase.

Carpal Tunnel Syndrome

This condition involves some sort of irritation of a nerve as it runs through the carpal tunnel (Figure 7.5). The exact cause is not fully understood and it is likely that there are several contributing factors. Examine your regular movements and positions to identify any obvious causative factors and address them as soon as possible. The symptoms of carpal tunnel syndrome can be varied, but may include a sensation of burning, tingling or numbness in some of the fingertips; these symptoms may wake you up during the night. The hand may also feel clumsy.

If you suspect that you may have carpal tunnel syndrome, we strongly recommend that you seek assessment by a qualified health or medical professional. We do not recommend any specific body-weight exercises to address this problem. Once you have been advised on your condition, and are safe to resume exercise, you may build up a generalised routine of body-weight exercise in order to develop your strength and flexibility at the wrist and forearm.

■ Body-weight Exercises for Improved Wrist Function

EXERCISE 7.5: FIST PUSH-UP SUPPORT

Target Area: Wrists, forearms
Sets: 3
Duration: 20 seconds
Rest: 30–45 seconds

LEVEL 2

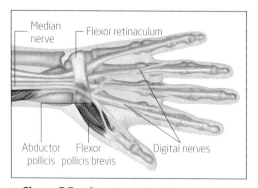

Figure 7.5. Carpal tunnel syndrome.

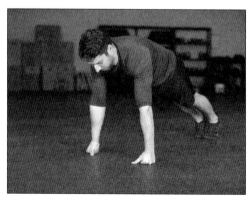

The fist push-up support is perfect for developing stability and strength in the wrists. It will expose any weakness you might have in wrist stability.

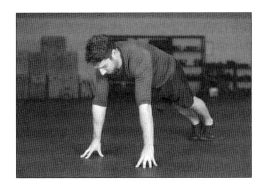

1. To perform the fist push-up support, place your fists on the ground, hands clenched and knuckles flat against the floor.
2. Balance on your toes so that you arrive in a push-up position. Make sure that your hands and forearms form a straight line.
3. Hold this position for the required time, and then rest. Repeat.

Teaching Points

If you are new to this type of exercise, you will no doubt be apprehensive about putting a lot of your body weight onto your wrists. If this is the case, and you are unsure of your ability, you can use a kneeling push-up position: instead of balancing on your toes, balance on your knees. A kneeling position will reduce the amount of body weight on the wrists, and allow you to gradually build up to the full version. Perform the exercise with your fists on towels or padded mats to increase comfort as necessary. Do not be a hero and cause unnecessary injury!

EXERCISE 7.6: FINGERTIP PUSH-UP SUPPORT

Target Area: Wrists, forearms
Sets: 3
Duration: 10–20 seconds
Rest: 30–45 seconds

LEVEL 3

If you are prepared for a physical challenge, consider the fingertip push-up support position; this is simply a push-up position in which your body weight is supported on the fingertips! This exercise helps hugely in building strength in the hands and forearms, and is a strong foundation for progressing to more complex body-weight exercises.

1. To perform the fingertip push-up support, place your hands on the ground, fingers splayed, with emphasis on the thumbs and index fingers.
2. Stretch your legs out behind you and assume a push-up position. Your shoulders, hips, knees and feet should form a straight line.
3. Hold this position for as long as possible, and then rest. Repeat.

Teaching Points

No doubt this movement will cause some issues if you do not have strong hands, or have weaknesses anywhere in the chain. To remedy this, perform the exercise in exactly the same way, but balance on the knees instead of the toes; this will reduce the amount of body weight being supported by the fingers, and will allow steady progression to the full version.

EXERCISE 7.7: FALSE-GRIP HANG

Target Area: Wrists, forearms
Sets: 3
Duration: 10–20 seconds
Rest: 30–45 seconds

LEVEL 3

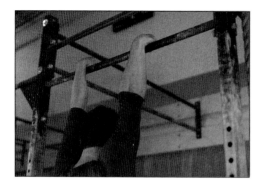

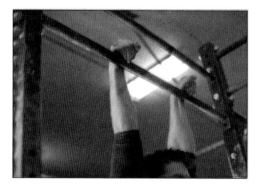

Strengthening the forearms is essential for developing injury resistance and rehabilitation in the wrists and elbows; the false-grip hang is excellent for doing this in the wrist flexors. The false grip itself is used in gymnastics to impart more control on the bar and on the still rings. Here, we can use it to our advantage in injury prevention and rehabilitation.

1. To perform the false-grip hang, stand on a box under a pull-up bar.
2. Wrap your hands around the bar and flex your hands so that the heels of your palms rest on top of the bar.
3. Keeping this position attempt to hang from the bar, allowing your elbows to straighten. If you have never done this before, you are likely to find it very difficult.
4. Hang for as long as possible, dropping off when your form starts to break down. Rest and repeat.

Teaching Points

The false-grip hang can be very difficult to master, and is included here for those of you wishing to develop higher levels of muscle strength and control. If this is you, then stick with this exercise. To make the movement easier, you can support your body weight with your legs; to do this, hang from the bar but keep your feet on the box or platform. Perform the hang, but support some of your weight with your legs, or with a single leg. As you become stronger, support less of your body weight with your legs.

EXERCISE 7.8: KNEELING INVERTED-WRIST PUSH-UP

Target Area: Wrists
Sets: 3
Reps: 5
Rest: 30–45 seconds

LEVEL 3

Once you have mastered supporting yourself on your wrists, it will be time to add a pushing element into the movement to make it even more challenging. This exercise will develop the wrist extensor muscles by using the inverted-wrist push-up support (Key Exercise 7.4). These push-ups are quite challenging, so only move on to them when you are ready.

1. To perform the kneeling inverted-wrist push-up, assume a kneeling push-up position but with the backs of your hands flat on the floor, fingers pointing inwards.
2. Keeping the backs of your hands pressed into the ground, start to lower yourself down to the floor by bending your elbows.
3. Keep going until your chest touches the floor (or as far as you can), and then push back up again until you reach the starting position. This counts as one repetition.

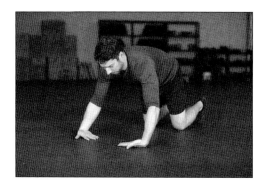

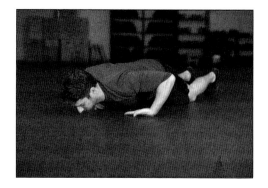

Teaching Points

If you find this exercise too difficult, it can be made easier. By bending at the hips, you can reduce the amount of weight put on the upper body, making the movement easier to complete. Another method is to place the hands on a raised platform; this will accomplish the same goal.

■ Goal Exercises for the Wrist

As with the other areas of the body, and in keeping with the other chapters in this book, we have developed a series of goal exercises that target the wrists, hands and forearms. These are a real test of wrist strength, mobility and flexibility, and will provide you with a benchmark of wrist function and resilience. These exercises can also be built into a full body workout to develop that bulletproof body.

GOAL EXERCISE 7.9: INVERTED-WRIST PUSH-UP

Primary Target Area: Wrists, forearms, shoulders
Sets: 3
Reps: 10
Rest: 30–45 seconds
LEVEL 3

The inverted-wrist push-up is an advanced exercise and should only be approached once you are familiar with the kneeling version of this exercise (Exercise 7.8). It is best to use an exercise mat here, and preferably one that is thick and offers a lot of cushioning.

1. To perform the inverted-wrist push-up, assume the inverted-wrist push-up support position. Ensure that your body is straight and you are balancing on your toes. Do not worry if you cannot maintain straight elbows.
2. Keeping the backs of your hands pressed into the ground, start to lower yourself down to the floor by bending your elbows. It helps to flex the fingers hard into the ground here, so as to keep the tension in the hands and ensure a solid platform.

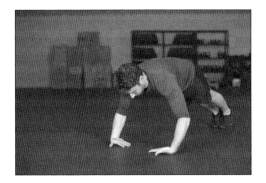

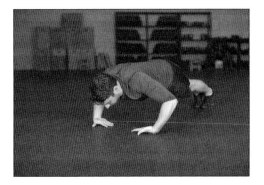

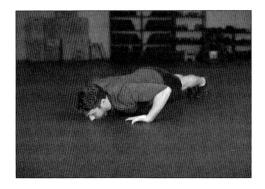

3. Keep going until your chest touches the floor (or as far as you can), and then push back up again until you reach the starting position. This counts as one repetition.

Teaching Points

This movement is very unusual for the uninitiated. Many people struggle with the pressure being placed upon the wrist, while others struggle with the flexibility required. Both of these issues can be solved by performing the kneeling version demonstrated previously (Exercise 7.8), and by an overall increase in strength. Proceed slowly and with care and you will develop in time.

If you need to make these easier, you should place your hands on a raised platform; this will take some of the weight off the upper body. As you progress, lower the height of the platform until you can perform these push-ups on level ground.

GOAL EXERCISE 7.10: FALSE-GRIP PULL-UP

Target Area: Wrists, forearms, elbows
Sets: 3
Reps: 3–5
Rest: 45–60 seconds   **LEVEL 3**

The false-grip hang (Exercise 7.7) is a great exercise, but we can make it more challenging by performing a pull-up in this position. This will put an extremely large demand on the muscles of the forearm, and help to build a very strong grip and bulletproof wrist flexors.

Once you are able to hang in a false grip for the required number of sets and repetitions, you can move on to the false-grip pull-up. This exercise is exactly what you would expect: the pull-up is performed with your hands in the false-grip position. It is especially difficult, and so do not be alarmed if it takes you some time to perfect it.

1. To perform the false-grip pull-up, assume the false-grip hang position.

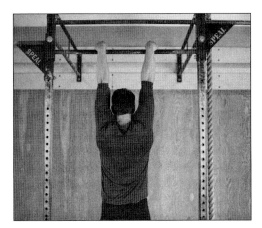

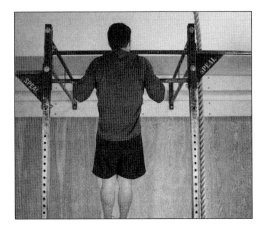

Teaching Points

As the false-grip pull-up is so tough, it is likely that you will not be able to perform a single repetition at first. To begin, start to pull as far as you can, using a reduced ROM. As you get stronger, the ROM you will be able to use will increase, and you will eventually be able to perform the movement properly.

GOAL EXERCISE 7.11: FIST-SUPPORTED TUCK PLANCHE

Target Area: Wrists, forearms, core muscles
Sets: 3
Reps: 5 seconds
Rest: 30–45 seconds

LEVEL 3

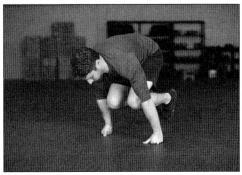

The planche is a gymnastic movement that is famous for its gravity-defying appearance. We can use a simplified version of it here to really strengthen the wrists. This is a high-level exercise, so only move on to this when ready.

2. Start to pull up towards the bar. You should aim to get your chin over the bar or your chest touching the bar.
3. At the top of the movement, hold for a second before lowering down to the starting position. This counts as one repetition.

1. To perform the fist-supported tuck planche, crouch down and place your fists on the ground, hands clenched tightly and knuckles against the floor.
2. Lean forwards so that most of your body weight is being supported by your fists.

3. Lift your feet off the ground and tuck them up into your chest, using your core muscles to do so.
4. Balance on your fists for as long as possible. Drop your feet down to the floor quickly if you feel the need or if you lose balance.

Teaching Points

Putting all of your body weight onto your wrists is difficult; if you are struggling with this movement, the best course of action is to raise your feet up for a second or so, and then drop them back down again. Do this to see how the exercise feels and to get an idea of how prepared you are for the movement.

In addition to the difficulty of supporting yourself on your wrists, the tuck planche will put a huge strain on your core and balance skills. It is quite natural for it to take a little time to build up the necessary strength and skill to perform the tuck planche, and so stick at it! Perform the exercise with the fists on a cushioned surface for comfort.

8

The Hip

◼ Introduction to the Hip

Powerful, deep and stable, the hip is one serious joint! It is a crucial weight-bearing structure with more natural mobility and stability than the knee, but without the complexity of the shoulder, which we encountered in Chapter 5. Whether you are moving between sitting and standing, climbing stairs or jumping into the air, it is the hip joint that powerfully levers the upper body over the lower limbs. We will now examine the crucial anatomy behind this mobile force generator, before exploring some common hip problems that could be alleviated with body-weight exercise.

◼ Functional Anatomy of the Hip

Passive Structures

In terms of bony anatomy, things do not come much simpler than the hip joint. The hip is a synovial, or freely mobile, joint that involves the bony hemisphere of the upper thigh bone (femur) sitting in the deep socket offered by the pelvic bones. As with all of the joints we have seen so far, the hip is reinforced with thick

ligaments and a joint capsule. The socket of the pelvis is deepened by a fibrous cartilage called the *labrum*, which forms a lip around the edge of the socket. The labrum can be a source of pain and dysfunction, so we will visit this briefly later on. As in the case of the shoulder (Chapter 5), the hip is a ball-and-socket joint, but unlike the shoulder it trades its mobility for weight-bearing ability. Movements available at the hip joint (Figure 8.1) are:

- Flexion
- Extension
- Abduction
- Adduction
- Internal rotation
- External rotation
- Circumduction (a combination of the above)

The final passive structure to mention here is the bursa. Bursae (plural) are fluid-filled sacs that are located around, or between, moving parts to reduce friction. There are two key bursae at the hip: one covers the greater trochanter, and the other is called the *iliopectineal bursa*, which is shown in Figure 8.2 along with the bony anatomy.

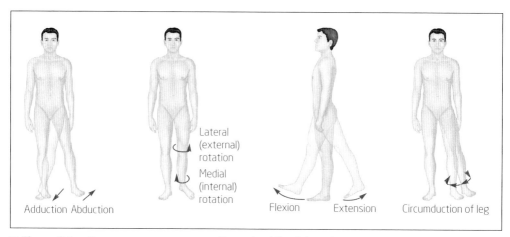

■ **Figure 8.1.** The many movements created by and stabilised through the hip joint.

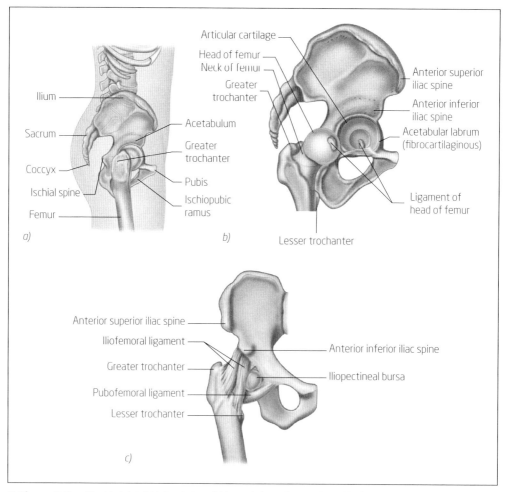

■ **Figure 8.2.** The hip joint: (a) lateral view; (b) lateral view of turned-out hip; (c) ligaments.

Unlike the shoulder joint, the hip joint trades mobility for weight-bearing ability.

Active Structures

As mentioned in previous chapters of this book, active structures are so called because they have a contracting function. This relates to the ability of muscles of the skeleton to shorten and pull on bones via their tendons, and is the basis of maintaining posture against gravity and of human movement.

The hip is an incredibly powerful joint owing to several of the muscles that act upon it. When rising from a chair, or squatting a weighted bar in the gym, it is the force generated by the hip muscles that allows the hip to straighten under load. Some of the many muscles found around the hip joint are shown in Figure 8.3. You will probably be familiar with many of their names from their common use in everyday language.

Some of the muscles in Figure 8.3 are grouped by their function rather than being named individually. You may be able to link these muscle groups to the movements of the hip discussed earlier in relation to passive structures; for example, *hip abduction* (taking the leg outwards and away from the centre line) is brought about by the contracting action of the *abductor muscles*.

Remember that the brain is thought to work in terms of movements rather than the activation of individual muscles. This is a key part of our message in aiming to promote functional and multi-muscle exercise; it is especially true in the lower limbs, where long muscles can cross two or more joints

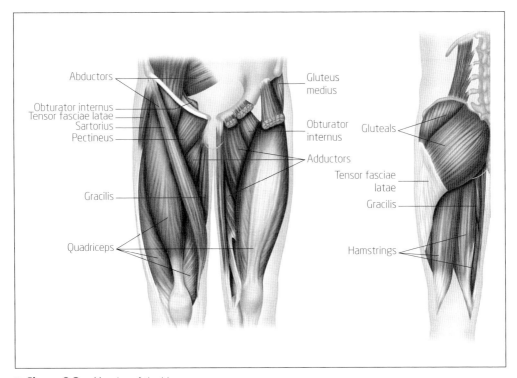

Abductors

Obturator internus
Tensor fasciae latae
Sartorius
Pectineus

Gracilis

Quadriceps

Gluteus medius

Obturator internus

Gluteals

Adductors

Tensor fasciae latae

Gracilis

Hamstrings

■ **Figure 8.3.** Muscles of the hip.

and act on both simultaneously under load. Look closely again at Figure 8.3 and note how the quadriceps spans the hip and the knee; although you may think of working the quadriceps by exercising the knee, you cannot discount the action of the hip in functional muscle training. The same can be said of the hamstrings, which are involved in extending (straightening) the hip and flexing (bending) the knee.

> **KEY POINT** *Functional exercises will use multiple muscles, often acting over more than one joint.*

Before we leave this discussion of the anatomy of the hip, it is worth pausing for a moment on the iliopsoas muscle. Figure 8.4 shows how this muscle is actually a combination of two muscles, the psoas and iliacus, which merge as they cross the front of the hip. Note how one of the iliopsoas muscles spans the lumbar spine and the

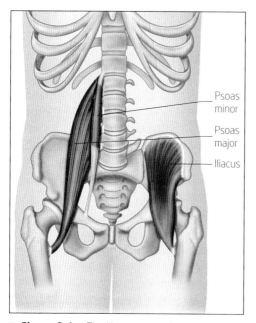

Psoas minor

Psoas major

Iliacus

■ **Figure 8.4.** The iliopsoas muscle.

front of the hip; now picture how sitting behind your desk or in your car all day could potentially shorten this muscle. Read on for key exercises to help reduce both lower back and hip pain!

■ Common Hip Dysfunction

From degenerative osteoarthritis to groin and hamstring strains, there are many reasons for pain in the hip region. These problems can potentially be alleviated or treated with movement-based therapies that focus on rehabilitating function, restoring pain-free movement and creating resilience. Even problematic bursae can respond positively to exercise by improving the movement around these fluid-filled structures and reducing some of the pressure upon them. Of all the joints discussed in this book, it is probably the hip joint that has the best capacity to improve through body-weight exercise.

One major consideration of hip function is quite simply that in most people the hip is not moved through anywhere near its full ROM. Although you can perhaps say the same of the shoulder, the hip especially lacks use as we become adults. Cast your mind back to your activities as a child: squatting and kneeling to play, running, jumping, climbing and kicking. It is often said by people with hip pain that they do not need therapy exercises for the hip because they are active – they walk everywhere. Walking is a wonderful exercise for general wellbeing and health; for mobilising the hip, however, it is not so good. Get up and walk around. How much range does your hip go through compared with what it could potentially achieve?

We will now explore some common hip problems, before focusing on targeted body-weight exercises.

Hip Joint Dysfunction

Degenerative osteoarthritis is not uncommon in the hip and is mostly seen above the age of 60. It can, however, occur in younger populations, and there are usually many reasons behind such development, including genetic factors, occupational or sporting overuse, previous fracture or trauma, or altered joint mechanics arising from leg length differences or from developmental abnormalities. If you are relatively young and have symptoms of joint arthritis, it is worth visiting a qualified health or medical professional for a thorough assessment.

KEY POINT *Strong contraction of the hip muscles during walking can produce an increase in load on the hip joint of up to four or five times one's body weight. This increased load might contribute to osteoarthritis at the hip joint.*

It has been suggested that the muscular forces around the hip can lead to the development of osteoarthritis. Strong contraction of the hip muscles during walking and standing on one leg is thought to produce an increase in load on the hip joint of up to four or five times one's body weight. This load increases with fast walking and running (I did say that walking was not a great exercise for hip pain); moreover, a stumble can create an impact load in excess of eight times the body's weight!

You will normally find that osteoarthritis causes a gradual onset of stiffness in the hip, which eventually becomes painful. We therefore offer Key Exercise 8.1 to mobilise the hip joint.

KEY EXERCISE 8.1: KNEE CIRCLE

Target Area: Hip mobility, shoulder and core strength
Sets: 2
Reps: 10 each leg
Rest: 10 seconds **LEVEL 1**

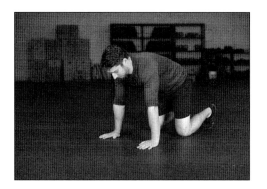

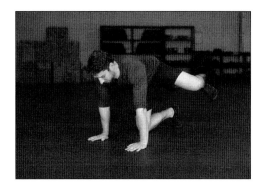

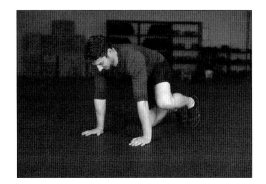

The knee circle is a great lower body mobility exercise that can be used to develop active hip mobility. The starting position gives a stability workout for the shoulders and core, while the muscle activity involved in performing the knee circles will also develop strength and endurance around the hip.

1. To perform the knee circle, position yourself on your hands and knees.
2. Raise one leg up to the side, taking the knee backwards before circling it forwards as far as you can. As mobility at the hip improves, you may be able to touch your planted arm with your circling knee. Return your knee to the starting position. Repeat on the other leg.

Teaching Point

Aim to draw a large arc with the knee. Use this exercise as a general warm-up exercise once your hip mobility increases. Progress to Exercise 8.8 (mountain climber) and Exercise 8.9 (frog hop).

Although it is not part of the bony structure at the hip, the labrum fibrocartilage sits within the hip joint. Damage to the labrum can be associated with osteoarthritis, or tears in the labrum may be caused by trauma, impingement between the bones of the hip joint, and joint laxity. Often, labrum-related problems cause symptoms including clicking, locking and a feeling of giving way at the hip; there may also be pinching pain when the hip is bent and the knee brought towards the opposite shoulder. In this case, we recommend assessment by a suitably qualified health or medical professional. If you have been cleared to exercise with this type of problem, try Key Exercise 8.2.

KEY EXERCISE 8.2: DEEP SQUAT POSITION

Target Area: Hips, knees, ankles
Sets: 3
Duration: 30 seconds
Rest: 20 seconds

LEVEL 1

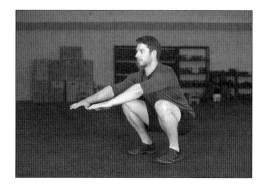

Being able to achieve a deep squat position is important in order to maintain a properly functioning lower body; when performed correctly, the exercise will increase mobility in the hips, knees and ankles. As a youngster, everyone is able to squat low and deep, but as age and sedentary lifestyles take over, this ability is lost. Getting back this ability is one the best things you can do to prevent injury and rehabilitate existing injuries.

1. To perform the deep squat position, place your feet flat on the floor, heels shoulder-width apart and your toes pointing slightly out.
2. Stretch your arms out in front of you and keep your eyes looking forwards, head and neck neutral.
3. Bend your knees, push your hips back and squat down as far as you can. Keep your lower back as straight as possible.

4. The position you are trying to achieve can be seen in the images; if you cannot get down this low, go as low as you can. Hold for 30 seconds, or as long as you are able to.

Teaching Points

Many people will struggle to get into this position at first, but there are a couple of things that can be done to make it more accessible. First, you can place your heels on a raised platform; this platform only needs to be 5cm high at most. Raising the heels in this way reduces the amount of stretch needed in the calves, allowing the knees to move further forwards, and allowing a deeper and lower squat.

Second, you can hold onto something with the hands and then lean back into the deep squat position. Suspension training systems or gymnastic rings are great for this, as you can support most of your weight and lean back; this allows you to get close to the proper position without having the hip mobility or ankle mobility needed to perform the movement without aid.

Hip Muscle/Tendon Strains

If you have recently had a trauma or strain of the muscles around the hip or thigh, we recommend that you have this assessed before trying any sort of physical exercise, including body-weight exercise. Such acute injuries are not the focus of this book; instead, we are concentrating on those niggles that you have had for some time, perhaps intermittently. These niggles may have started as a sudden strain, or perhaps even resulted from gradual overuse, but for whatever reason have not fully settled and have left you with some area of weakness or physical vulnerability.

It is time to give nature some direction and bulletproof these problematic areas with body-weight exercise!

The most common hip and thigh muscle problems tend to include the hamstrings, quadriceps and adductors (inner thigh), although any muscle can be subject to strain or direct trauma. The good news is that we do not need to isolate these muscles. Keep it functional and you should be able to find that weakness and turn it into a strength.

As the hamstrings and quadriceps (rectus femoris) cross both the hip and the knee, there is a greater potential for overuse or sudden strain. Poor posture, poor physical conditioning, inadequate warm-up prior to rapid movements, and muscle fatigue have been described as precipitating factors. Studies have found that muscle imbalances between the hamstrings and quadriceps can increase the risk of hamstring injury by four to five times. Old muscle injuries may have healed after a period of rest, but you could have been left with a tight or short muscle that is vulnerable to re-injury. There is evidence to suggest that graded stretching should be part of your rehabilitation. Thorough functional stretching should also be part of your injury prevention toolkit. Try Key Exercises 8.3 and 8.4 for starters.

KEY EXERCISE 8.3: HAMSTRING STRETCH

Target Area: Hip mobility, hamstring flexibility
Sets: 3
Duration: 20 seconds each leg
Rest: 20 seconds

LEVEL 1

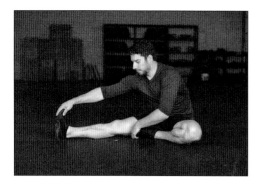

The hamstrings can be painful in themselves but can also contribute to the lower back pain discussed in Chapter 11 of this book; the reason for this is that the flexibility of the hamstrings dictates the ability of the lower back, pelvis, hip and knee to move freely. Touching the toes and being able to close the hips is a generally a good indicator of hamstring flexibility, although you may feel the restriction in your lower back.

1. To perform the hamstring stretch, sit down on the floor with one leg out in front of you. Tuck your other leg into your buttocks and lay it flat on the floor.
2. Reach forwards and bend at the hips, aiming to keep your back straight. You should feel the stretch in the back of the thigh in the straight leg.
3. Move forwards until you feel a good stretch in the hamstrings. Hold for 20 seconds, change legs and repeat.

Teaching Points

Most people do not stretch their hamstrings enough, even if they are following a training program to increase their flexibility; this is because many people sit for long periods in their daily lives and therefore do not experience a regular functional stretch. The act of sitting shortens and reduces the flexibility of the hamstrings for the simple reason that the sitting

position requires the knee joint to be flexed while the pelvis is tilted backwards. If this applies to you, we recommend spending a little more time stretching your hamstrings with the body-weight winner Key Exercise 8.4.

KEY EXERCISE 8.4: GROIN STRETCH

Target Area: Hips, adductors, hamstrings, lower back
Sets: 3
Duration: 20 seconds
Rest: 20 seconds

LEVEL 1

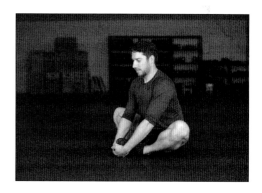

In addition to building strength in the hips, it is a very good idea to make sure that they are flexible enough to reduce the risk of strain. The groin stretch presented here is excellent for increasing the flexibility of the adductor muscles, which are the long muscles on the insides of the thighs.

1. To perform the groin stretch, sit down with the soles of your feet together. Use your hands to pull your feet as close to your buttocks as possible. If you find that the bony parts on the outer side of each ankle feel uncomfortable, cushion them with a hand towel.

2. Sit up straight and attempt to bring your knees as low to the floor as possible. You can use the muscles on the outsides of your legs to pull your knees down, or you can simply push on them with your arms or hands. Hold this position for 20 seconds.

Teaching Points

To increase the stretch even further, you can lean forwards and try to pull your chest towards your feet; this will also help to stretch some of the gluteal muscles and the lower back. A good practice is to try to get your forearms flat against the floor. This exercise will target multiple muscles in the hip and thigh.

Hip Bursa Dysfunction

Direct trauma to the hip may cause the bursae to swell and become painful, but more often they tend to give pain because of overuse or excessive friction. There are several bursae around the hip, with at least four of them situated between the gluteal muscles. These fluid-filled bags allow moving structures to slide over each other without excessive friction; however, altered joint mechanics, postural stress and muscle imbalances can create so much pressure that the bursae become excessively loaded.

The psoas bursa lies beneath the iliopsoas muscle, which we will discuss below, whereas the trochanteric bursa (Figure 8.5) separates the gluteus maximus muscle from the bony point on the outside of your hip. As mentioned above, the numerous gluteal bursae provide padding for the gluteal muscles. By correcting muscle imbalances in these areas, you can potentially restore the normal load and functioning of the hip bursae, allowing nature to do its thing and settle any bursal irritation over the following weeks. Key Exercise 8.5 is recommended

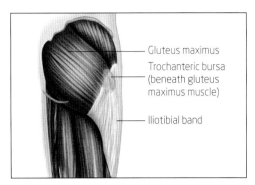

Gluteus maximus

Trochanteric bursa (beneath gluteus maximus muscle)

Iliotibial band

■ **Figure 8.5.** Trochanteric bursa.

for stretching the glutes (gluteal or buttock muscles).

KEY EXERCISE 8.5: GLUTE STRETCH

Target Area: Hips, glutes
Sets: 3
Duration: 20 seconds each leg
Rest: 20 seconds   LEVEL 1

The glutes are the largest and most powerful muscles in the body; it is therefore important to stretch them to maintain performance

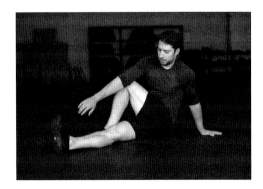

in running, jumping and other lower body movements. In addition, tightness here can inhibit free movement of the hips, causing other issues further down the line. As with the hamstrings, it is important to keep the glutes functioning correctly, as they power many lower body movements.

1. To perform the glute stretch, sit down with one leg straight and the other leg bent.
2. Now place the foot of the bent leg on the outside of the knee of the straight leg.
3. Push the bent knee towards your straight leg until you feel the stretch in your glute. Keep your hips as square as possible.
4. Hold this position for 20 seconds, change legs and repeat.

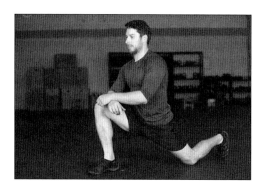

Iliopsoas Syndrome/Dysfunction

As discussed above, the iliopsoas muscle has a tendon that crosses the front of the hip, with the psoas bursa sitting between the tendon and the hip joint. In iliopsoas syndrome, there may be increased friction and pressure on the bursa, causing bursitis, or there may be inflammation of the iliopsoas tendon. As a result of modern sedentary postures, there may even be long-term shortening of the iliopsoas muscle, altering the hip joint mechanics and placing stress on the lumbar spine. Hip movements may be restricted and painful, and there may even be a clicking or snapping sensation as the taught tendon moves over surrounding structures. All of these things can cause pain. If you address the primary problem of a shortened/contracted iliopsoas muscle, you will in turn probably restore normal hip and spine movements and offload the tendon and bursa. See how you get on with Key Exercise 8.6.

KEY EXERCISE 8.6: HIP FLEXOR STRETCH

Target Area: Hip flexors, lumbar spine
Sets: 3
Duration: 20 seconds each leg
Rest: 20 seconds

LEVEL 1

The hip flexor stretch, when done properly and with patience, may well be the best exercise you ever do for hip and lower back pain. The hip flexors include the iliopsoas and the rectus femoris (quadriceps), and so together these muscles span from the lumbar spine to below the knee joint! When you do the stretch, remember this fact and maintain a good posture of your trunk. Modern sedentary lifestyles make this area prone to poor function; keeping the hip flexor muscles flexible can therefore be key to reducing injury risk at the hip and lower back.

1. To perform the hip flexor stretch, assume a kneeling position with one leg in front of you. Keep your torso upright.
2. Lean forwards, aiming to push the hips forwards and down. Rest your arms on your front leg to aid balance.
3. You should feel a stretch at the top of your rear leg, at the front of the straight hip, and possibly deep in your back. If you do not, gently contract your glute muscles to push the hip forwards and increase the stretch. Hold this position for 20 seconds, change sides and repeat.

Teaching Points

The hip flexor stretch is one that should progress fairly rapidly, but some readers may still need to make it a little easier to manage.

If you wish to make the exercise easier, move the knee and the foot closer together.

If you are looking to increase the stretch, you can drive the hip further forwards, or you can grab your rear foot and pull it up to your buttocks to stretch the quadriceps (rectus femoris). For an increased stretch of the iliopsoas, take the arm on the side being stretched and reach it over your head, flexing your trunk away from the stretch.

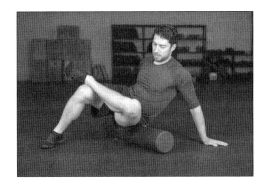

Body-weight Exercises for Improved Hip Function

EXERCISE 8.7: PIRIFORMIS FOAM ROLL AND STRETCH

Target Area: Hips
Sets: 3
Duration: 20–30 seconds each leg
Rest: 30 seconds   **LEVEL 2**

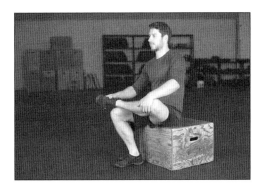

Incorporating squatting and lunging movements into your training can increase the tightness and irritation of the piriformis, a muscle deep in the buttock. If the piriformis muscle becomes tight, it can manifest itself with sciatica-like symptoms in the affected area. To take care of this problem, we can foam roll the piriformis; this can be performed with either a foam roller or a tennis ball. Beware – this exercise can be uncomfortable, so go slowly at first!

1. To foam roll and stretch your piriformis, sit down and place your right foot on the left knee, as if you were going to cross your legs.
2. Now sit directly on the foam roller with the piriformis. You will know if you are on the right spot, as it should feel tender. It may even feel knotted deep in the buttock.
3. Roll over the tight spot slowly for 20–30 seconds, and then change legs and repeat.
4. Once you have foam rolled both sides, you should perform a static stretch. To do this, sit on a chair with one foot flat on the floor and your knee at 90 degrees.
5. Place your free foot on the knee of the working leg, and push down on the knee of the free foot. You will feel the stretch in the piriformis/deep buttock. Keep the torso upright and breathe deeply. Hold the stretch for 20 seconds, and then change sides and repeat.

Teaching Points

Piriformis foam rolling can be a sore process. This is expected, but it is best to start with a soft foam roller; then, as you become more experienced, move to firmer foam rollers. You can also use a tennis ball (progressing to a baseball or a cricket ball) to really get into the muscle; this is recommended for experienced exercisers only, as the pain can be quite intense.

EXERCISE 8.8: MOUNTAIN CLIMBER

Target Area: Hips
Sets: 3
Reps: 10 each leg
Rest: 30 seconds

LEVEL 2

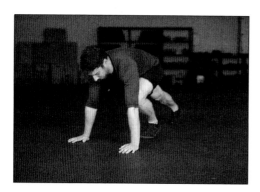

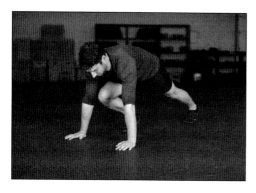

Climb every mountain! The mountain climber is a superb all-round exercise that is normally performed as a cardiovascular exercise in boot camps or group exercise classes. With some alterations, however, it can be very good for increasing strength and mobility in the hips. The exercise is a little more vigorous than the stretches in this chapter, so approach it with care if you are new to physical training.

1. To perform the mountain climber, assume a push-up position. Stretch one leg out behind you and place the other leg as close to the outside of your hand as possible.
2. Keeping your arms straight. jump both feet into the air and change them over so that the rear foot comes to the front and the front foot goes to the rear.
3. Repeat for 10 repetitions each leg, i.e. 20 repetitions in total, with each individual jump counting as a single repetition.

Teaching Points

The aim of this exercise is to increase strength and mobility in the hips; therefore, do not worry about trying to do the repetitions as fast as possible. Slow, controlled movement is the best course of action here. It may take you some time to build up the mobility in your hips to be able to achieve the ROM shown in the images. In this case, you could step the bent leg back along the straight leg, and then step the other leg in towards the arms. Keep at it and the flexibility will come!

EXERCISE 8.9: FROG HOP

Target Area: Hips
Sets: 3
Reps: 10
Rest: 30 seconds

LEVEL 2

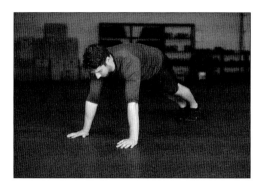

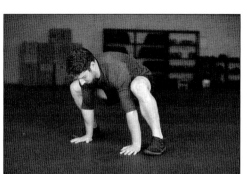

The frog hop can be a progression from the mountain climber if you want to add an aerobic emphasis, but it can also be done in a controlled way to focus on hip mobility and strength. The frog hop is included here as a dynamic movement, which differs from the static stretches and foam rolling seen previously.

1. To perform the frog hop, assume a push-up position. Your hands should be flat on the floor, shoulder-width apart.
2. From here, jump both feet forwards. You should be aiming to get them to land on the outside of your hands. If you do not have the mobility to do this, go as far forward as you can.
3. Pause for a second, and then jump your feet backwards so that you arrive back in the push-up position. This counts as one repetition.

Teaching Points

To make the frog hop easier, you can place your hands on a platform or step of some sort. Raising the hands in this way will allow you to develop the hip flexibility and mobility gradually, which is especially useful if you have problems or an injury in this area. Over time, you can move the hands closer to the ground.

Progression/Variation

To progress the frog hop to become more of an all-over conditioning exercise, and to get more dynamic mobility at the hips and lower back, try travelling from the frog position by leading with your arms and hopping forwards in a straight line. Each time you jump to your arms, place them out in front of you again and repeat the process of hopping into your arms. This variation can also be performed backwards by pushing through the arms and then hopping the legs backwards, before bringing the arms back to meet the legs and repeating.

KEY POINT *The frog hop is a personal favourite of ours and has given good results with chronic hip and lower back stiffness and pain. Build up slowly, though!*

■ Goal Exercises for the Hips

As with the other chapters of this book, we present some goal exercises; these will build hip strength and mobility and also act as a test of your physical condition. The movements actually build on the movements discussed previously, and include a greater ROM and a greater use of strength.

GOAL EXERCISE 8.10: BODY-WEIGHT SQUAT

Target Area: Hips, knees, ankles
Sets: 3
Reps: 10–20
Rest: 30–45 seconds

LEVEL 1

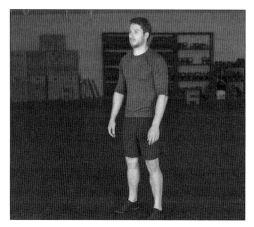

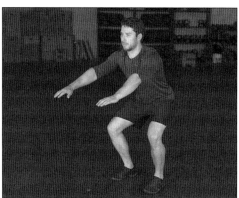

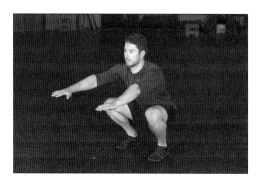

The body-weight squat is perhaps the most useful lower body exercise with regard to strength and mobility; this is because it is a compound movement. A *compound movement* is one which involves many joints and muscle groups all working in unison, which is what contributes to the potential strength gains and increases in usable mobility. This is the essence of developing a bulletproof body.

1. To perform the body-weight squat, stand with your feet shoulder-width apart, toes pointing out at a slight angle.
2. Push your hips back and bend the knees, beginning the squat. Allow your arms to reach forwards to aid balance.
3. Keep descending, forcing the knees out so that they follow the line made by your toes.
4. Keep the lower back straight and tight, and the head and eyes neutral and looking forwards.
5. Descend as far as your strength and mobility allow: this is the bottom part of the squat. Ideally, you should be aiming to reach the depth shown in the images.
6. Pause for a second, and then return to a standing position. This counts as one repetition.

Teaching Points

The body-weight squat looks simple but can take a while to perform perfectly. In addition to the strength required, mobility is the aspect that will cause issues for most people. The deep squat position (Key Exercise 8.2) will help with this, as will the various lower body stretches in this chapter.

You may be restricted by mobility of the ankle joint. To solve this problem, your heels can be placed on a very small platform, 2.5cm or so in height; you can use anything sturdy and solid for this, as long as the object does not move. This method raises the heels and requires less ankle flexibility, which will allow you to drop lower into the squat while still maintaining proper form. As you progress, simply take away the platform under the heels, and transition to the full movement.

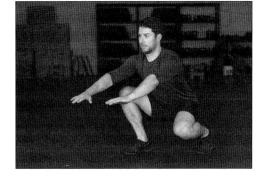

GOAL EXERCISE 8.11: DUCK WALK

Target Area: Hips
Sets: 3
Reps: 10–20 steps
Rest: 30–45 seconds   **LEVEL 3**

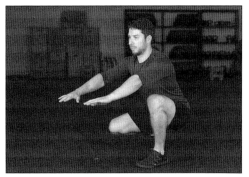

The duck walk is a great exercise for testing the mobility and strength of the hips; it can be thought of as a natural progression of the deep squat position (Key Exercise 8.2). The duck walk is exactly what it sounds like: a moving exercise in which the aim is to keep the buttocks as low to the ground as possible, while moving the hips through a large ROM. In other words, it involves walking like a duck!

1. To perform the duck walk, assume a deep squat position. Place the arms wherever they feel comfortable, and in a position where they can aid balance.
2. Without rising up too much, take a step forwards. The distance will need to be small in order to avoid raising the hips into the air.
3. As you place the front foot down, allow the rear heel to rise. Once you are settled on the front foot, take a step forwards with the other foot. You may have to rotate the hips slightly to do this.
4. Keep going for the required number of steps, rest and repeat.

Teaching Points

If you cannot perform the duck walk as outlined, simply squat down as low as your mobility allows and then walk in this position. As your strength and mobility increase, you should be able to drop the hips lower and lower until you can perform the movement as demonstrated. You can also spend more time practising the deep squat position to build up the flexibility in your hips.

9

The Knee

■ Introduction to the Knee

Unlike the deep-fitting hip joint, the knee joint lacks bony stability. In the knee, the bulbous lower end of the thighbone sits on a flat bony shelf offered by the upper end of the shinbone. When you stand from a seated position, the moving thighbone rolls forwards over the upper shinbone while also sliding backwards. With no bony limit to the amount of sliding, it is down to the numerous ligaments in the knee to stop one bone sliding free of the other. When you kick a football, the reverse action occurs, with the shinbone rolling and sliding forwards on the thighbone. Once again, the ligaments of the knee ensure that the lower leg does not follow the ball as it flies through the air.

The knee joint is truly a structure that is greater than the sum of its parts. It is much more than a collection of bones and ligaments: in this chapter, we outline the other numerous structures that make the knee unique, but also susceptible to injury.

■ Functional Anatomy of the Knee

Passive Structures

The knee allows the transmission of weight from the thigh to the lower leg, while facilitating movement during functions such as walking, running and jumping. Most of this movement occurs at a specific joint in the knee, where the femur (thigh bone) meets the tibia (shin bone). There is also another very important joint at the knee, created where the femur joins the patella (knee cap). The relationship of these joints and their bones can be seen in Figure 9.1. You will also see that the thinner fibula bone creates a third, less mobile, joint with the tibia.

The patellofemoral joint allows the patella to ride over the lower femur as the knee flexes and extends, and also plays a role in distributing the powerful forces created by the muscles at the front of the knee. The 'true' knee joint, between the tibia and the femur, is where the more familiar functions of the knee are permitted. As a hinge joint, it facilitates flexion and extension, allowing you to squat, sit, stand and more. The limitation to these movements comes not

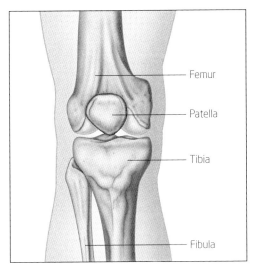

■ **Figure 9.1.** Bones of the knee, right leg, anterior view.

injured structures in the knee and will be discussed more specifically later in this chapter.

The otherwise flat top of the tibia is deepened by two ring-like cartilage structures that provide some stability and cushioning to the knee joint. These cartilages are known as the *menisci* (plural), illustrated in Figure 9.2(b), and these too can be susceptible to injury, as we shall see later in this chapter.

> **KEY POINT** *The moveable knee is made up of two main joints: one between the shin and the thighbone, and one between the kneecap and the thighbone.*

from the bony shape of the knee joint, but from the ligaments that bind the bones and restrain further range. Figure 9.2(a) identifies the main ligaments of the knee.

The ligaments of the knee include the lateral collateral ligament (LCL) and medial collateral ligament (MCL), as well as the more familiar cruciate ligaments – the anterior cruciate ligament (ACL) and the posterior cruciate ligament (PCL). These are commonly

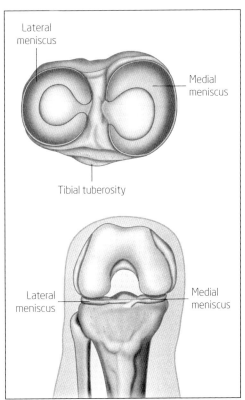

■ **Figure 9.2b.** The menisci (right leg, anterior view) with bird's eye view inset.

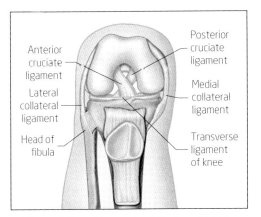

■ **Figure 9.2a.** Ligaments of the knee (right leg, anterior view, with knee bent at 90 degrees).

The knee is reported to have between 11 and 14 bursae. These fluid-filled sacs can be an extension of the joint capsule and its lubricating fluid; they are located around the mobile structures of the knee joint to prevent friction between the joint's moving parts. The bursae can, however, be subjected to excessive friction and pressure and consequently become problematic, as we shall see later in this chapter.

Active Structures

The knee is crossed by tendons or tendon-like structures on all four sides, which further act to stabilise the lower femur on the flat upper tibia. No fewer than 12 muscles provide support to the knee, and when they contract they will contribute to the movement available here. Figure 9.3 shows several of these muscles. You may recognise some of the

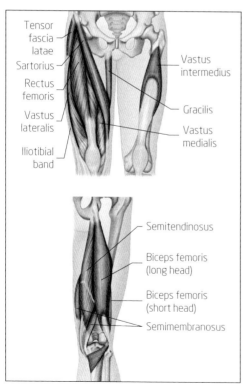

■ **Figure 9.3.** Muscles of the knee.

names of the muscles that make up the muscle groups of the hamstrings and quadriceps. As a general rule, those muscles passing the front of the knee will extend the joint when they contract, while those passing behind the centre line of the joint will cause it to flex.

It is not just the knee joint being acted upon by some of the muscles in Figure 9.3. As we have seen in the upper limbs elsewhere in this book, several long muscles span two or more joints, and those crossing the knee are no exception. Some of these begin above the hip joint and pass to just below the knee. Others, such as the gastrocnemius and plantaris, originate just above the knee and descend to below the ankle (see Chapter 10). Two-joint muscles have a dual role to play at any given time; they can therefore be more susceptible to injury in terms of strains or chronic stress. These muscles may be stabilising one joint while moving the other, stabilising both joints simultaneously against another force, or moving both joints at the same time. Body-weight exercises are therefore ideal for injury-proofing the muscles crossing the knee by developing multi-joint activity and stability.

> **KEY POINT** *As a general rule, those muscles passing the front of the knee will extend the joint, while those passing behind the centre line of the joint will cause it to flex.*

The muscles of the knee merge into tendons before anchoring at their bony destination. There are several tendons crossing the knee: these include the three long tendons of the hamstring group, and the single patellar ligament of the quadriceps group. In addition to these more familiar tendons, we will also consider the iliotibial band (ITB) on the outer aspect of the knee, and the three-pronged ('goose-foot') tendon structure on the inner aspect of the knee. These are all points of potential injury or weakness, and will therefore be reviewed in relation to specific knee problems.

■ Common Knee Dysfunction

During childhood, it would have been commonplace for your knees to fully flex and extend regularly throughout the day. As we become adults, however, the knee tends to be subjected to less ROM, which means that some parts of the joint become less loaded, stretched and lubricated over time. There may now be valid reasons why you are no longer able to squat, kneel or sit cross-legged, but it may also be that these movements are no longer accessible to you because you have not 'trained' for them in a while. In this way, you become trapped in a cycle of stiffness and pain that can lock you into a world of reduced function.

> **KEY POINT** *During childhood, it would have been commonplace for your knees to fully flex and extend throughout the day, receiving increased load, more movement and better lubrication.*

We will explore how body-weight exercises might be used to break the cycle of knee pain and reduced function, allowing you to live a fuller and freer life of movement.

Knee Joint Arthritis

The knee is the most common site in the body for osteoarthritis: it is estimated that, at the time of writing, about 18% of the population of England aged 45 and over have osteoarthritis of the knee. Not all knee osteoarthritis, however, is painful or restrictive. In the USA, around 12% of adults aged 65 or over have problematic knee osteoarthritis. Unless the arthritis is advanced or severe (relatively few cases in people under 65 years of age), there is a wonder treatment to help manage the pain, stiffness and reduced function in the knee. It is a treatment that has support from the research literature, and is emphasised in clinical guidelines in the UK and elsewhere in the world. It is a treatment known as 'exercise'! That's right, *exercise*. When tailored to your own needs, it can help reduce and manage some of the problems associated with knee arthritis. Before we go on to look at some suitable body-weight exercises for an arthritic knee, let us first consider briefly the nature of osteoarthritis.

> **KEY POINT** *There exists a wonder treatment for managing knee osteoarthritis that is well supported by research evidence. It is called 'exercise'!*

Osteoarthritis is very different from rheumatoid arthritis, and the management of the two conditions will differ accordingly. If you are unsure which condition you are experiencing, we suggest you are reviewed by a medical or health professional. Osteoarthritis is a condition that affects your joints; through mostly 'wear-and-tear' damage, the smooth cartilage on the ends of the bones becomes patchy, thin and roughened. The damaged cartilage can irritate the joint from time to time, causing it to swell. The joint may also become thickened, or lose its original shape over time as the body compensates with new bone growth. Osteoarthritis tends to flare and settle in the joints intermittently. Seek medical or health care reassurance for the flare-ups; otherwise, we recommend managing the settled osteoarthritic knee with tailored exercise. Body-weight exercise can form part of this management plan, and we recommend Key Exercise 9.1.

KEY EXERCISE 9.1: SQUAT

Target Area: Knees, hips
Sets: 3
Reps: 5–20
Rest: 45 seconds

LEVEL 1

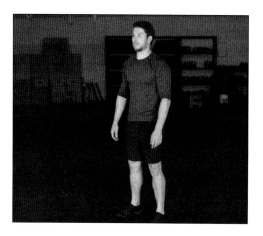

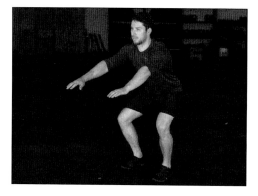

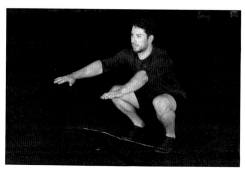

The squat is a fundamental lower body exercise requiring nothing more than good form and your body weight to get real results. Using a hip drive technique, the knees and hips are brought into extension from deep flexion using the muscles we have discussed previously. This exercise is included here because it will promote knee flexion, which is often first affected in knee osteoarthritis, and will develop the muscles around the knee that can become wasted.

1. To perform the squat, stand with heels shoulder-width apart and hands folded across your chest or out in front of you. Keep your toes pointed forwards or out-turned by about 30 degrees, whichever is most comfortable for you.
2. Bend at the knees, keeping your back straight and your head up with your eyes looking forwards. Push your hips back and downwards at the same time. As you descend, allow your knees to fall outwards slightly so that the hips can fall between them. Do not allow your knees to move forward of your toes. Keep your feet flat.
3. Squat down as low as your mobility and ability allow. As you progress with ROM and strength, your hips may sit lower than your knees. It takes time, though, so persevere.
4. From this bottom position, drive your hips up and forwards and gradually extend your knee to develop the inner quadriceps muscle bulk.

Teaching Points

This is a complex movement with lots going on. Good form is essential here, so pay attention to your body position and do not overstress your knees too soon. As strength and mobility improve, you can make the squat deeper.

Also recommended: Key Exercise 8.2 (deep squat position).

Patellofemoral Pain Syndrome

Patellofemoral pain syndrome (or PFPS for short) is a condition characterised by pain around the front of the knee (Figure 9.4). The pain may be felt under the kneecap, but can often be a vague ache around the knee. The problem mostly originates from the area where the back of the patella (knee cap) makes contact with the lower end of the femur (thigh bone). The diagnosis is usually made when other more specific problems have been ruled out. If you are unsure, see a medical or health or professional.

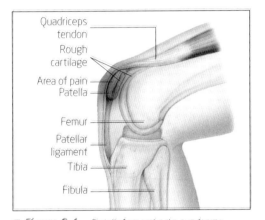

■ **Figure 9.4.** Patellofemoral pain syndrome.

The cause of PFPS is usually some form of increased or excessive pressure on the patellofemoral joint of the knee. This abnormal pressure may be due to muscle imbalances, tight soft-tissue structures, unaccustomed physical activity, or biomechanical pressures from changes to lower-limb posture.

First-line treatment involves relative rest from the initial cause, followed by exercise therapy to include stretching and strengthening exercises for the legs and hips/buttocks. Key Exercise 9.2 should definitely be in your routine, along with a few other essential exercises that we also recommend.

KEY EXERCISE 9.2: QUADRICEPS STRETCH

Target Area: Knees, quadriceps muscles
Sets: 3
Duration: 20–30 seconds each leg
Rest: 20 seconds   LEVEL 1

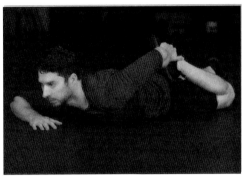

It is important to maintain mobility and muscular flexibility around the knee to relieve some pressure on the patellofemoral joint. The quadriceps stretch maintains and increases flexibility in the front of the thigh.

1. To perform the quadriceps stretch, lie face down. Position one forearm on the ground so that your chest and shoulders are slightly raised.
2. Keep one leg straight and bring the heel of the other leg up to your buttocks. Grab the bent leg with your free hand.
3. Pull your foot to your buttocks, making sure to keep your leg square onto your hips. Pull your foot until you feel a stretch in your quadriceps at the front of your thigh. This should be a mildly uncomfortable position, but never painful.
4. Hold this position for 20–30 seconds, and then change legs and repeat.

Teaching Points

If you do have flexibility issues around the front of the knee, this stretch is a must.

Work within your limits, and then increase the ROM over time.

Also recommended: Key Exercise 8.3 (hamstring stretch), Key Exercise 8.4 (groin stretch), Key Exercise 8.6 (hip flexor stretch).

Knee Ligament Injury

As we outlined earlier in this chapter, there are four main ligaments that bind the knee and help prevent excessive movement at this joint: these are the ACL, PCL, MCL

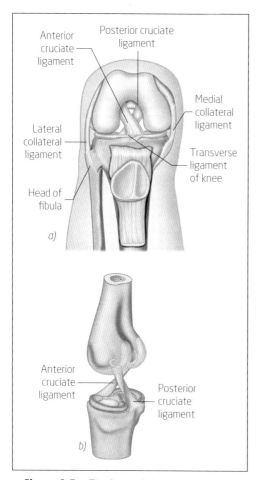

and LCL (Figure 9.5). The cruciates sit inside the knee joint and roughly cross each other from the front to the back (cruciate = cross-shaped).

Crudely speaking, the ACL and PCL prevent excessive forwards-backwards movement of the shinbone under the thighbone. These two ligaments also offer some rotational support, so any injury involving rotation or hyperextension (over-straightening) of the knee may traumatise them. Because of the mechanism of injury common to the knee, it is most likely to be the ACL that is damaged. If you are experiencing an acute injury, we recommend that a health or medical professional assesses you. If you have an ongoing degree of instability in the knee and have been told that you do not require surgical repair, add Key Exercise 9.3 to your routine. If you do not have a history of ACL injury but instead want to injury-proof this ligament, you should definitely work on this exercise.

KEY EXERCISE 9.3: GYM BALL HAMSTRING CURL

Target Area: Knees, hamstrings
Sets: 3
Reps: 10
Rest: 20 seconds

LEVEL 2

This exercise requires a gym (Swiss) ball, but can also be done (but with more difficulty) using a soccer ball or basketball. The gym ball hamstring curl develops the ability of the hamstring muscles to lengthen under load and control the extension of the knee. It also develops active stability in the knee by creating a less stable base.

■ **Figure 9.5.** The four main knee ligaments. (a) right leg, anterior view; (b) right leg, posterior view.

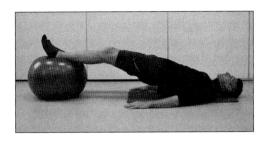

can even use a basketball or similar. Vary the speed of the movement to develop a more dynamic extension of the knee. If you want a real challenge, work towards performing the exercise one leg at a time!

Also recommended: Exercise 11.14 (bridge).

The collateral ligaments sit along either side of the joint and contribute to stability on the inner and outer aspects of the joint. The LCL is shorter and thicker, and sits slightly away from the joint; the MCL is thinner and flatter, sits close to the side of the joint and has a common mechanism of injury, making it prone to trauma. If you have a chronic instability at the MCL, or want to make this ligament resilient to future injury, try Key Exercise 9.4.

1. Lie on your back with straight legs and place your heels up onto a gym ball. Use your glutes and hamstrings to raise your buttocks off the floor. Some of your weight will now be resting onto the back of the shoulders. Do not strain your head or neck. Work on controlling stability here, as the ball will want to move side to side in the starting position. Place your hands and arms flat on the floor either side of you for increased stability.
2. Keeping shoulders and arms firmly in contact with the floor, begin to roll the ball towards your buttocks by 'curling' your hamstrings. Work hard on maintaining stability and balance as you draw the ball under your bent knees.
3. Slowly roll the ball back to the starting position, feeling the hamstrings lengthen under the strain. As you approach the starting position again, do not allow your knees to snap into extension. This should be a controlled return movement. Repeat.

Teaching Points

Play around with different-size gym balls to change the stability aspect. As suggested, you

KEY EXERCISE 9.4: V-UP WITH BALL SQUEEZE

Target Area: Core and adductor muscles
Sets: 3
Reps: 5–10
Rest: 30 seconds

LEVEL 3

The V-up is a combination of a sit-up and a leg extension, but when you add a ball to the mix it takes on a different challenge. With the use of a football or similar, the aim here is to apply a gentle squeeze on the ball by the feet; this puts a slight stress on the inner knee to activate the adductor muscles. As the knee then moves through flexion and extension, this activation is maintained to develop support around the MCL.

1. Lie on your back with a ball held between both feet.

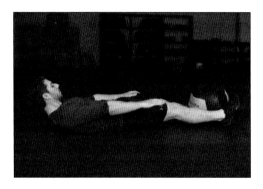

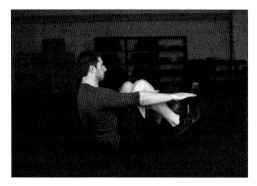

Also recommended: Exercise 11.10 (side plank).

Knee Cartilage Dysfunction

There are two types of cartilage found in the knee joint: 1) smooth 'articular' cartilage, which covers the joining surfaces of bones and reduces the friction of joint movement; and 2) fibrous cartilage, which makes up the crescent-shaped ('sickle-moon') menisci. Each meniscus sits on top of the shinbone and cushions the impact of the lower thighbone. The cartilaginous menisci can degenerate and fray with time and use, leading to niggles in later life. In younger life, they may be subject to outright tears, usually resulting from excessive rotational movements (Figure 9.6).

2. Brace your core and raise your upper back off the floor. Keeps your arms by your sides to reduce the lever strain on your trunk.
3. Raise your torso further by using your abdominal muscles. Simultaneously bend your knees and raise them towards your chest. Keep hold of the ball between your feet!
4. Once your chest and knees have almost met in the middle, hold this position momentarily before slowly returning to the starting position. Remember, the aim is to maintain the squeeze on the ball as the knees move through the range. Repeat.

Teaching Points

If the core aspect of this exercise is too difficult, keep your back flat on the floor and simply extend and return your feet while keeping hold of the ball. For more of a challenge, use a weighted ball and balls of different sizes.

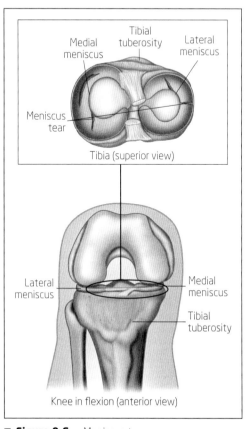

■ **Figure 9.6.** Meniscus tear.

As the medial (inner) meniscus bears more load and has less rotational freedom it is most likely to be injured.

If you have been advised by a health professional to exercise the knee to deal with this problem, or you want to reduce your injury risk here, give Key Exercise 9.5 a go.

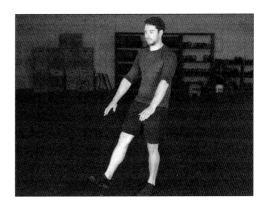

KEY EXERCISE 9.5: SINGLE-LEG SQUAT

Target Area: Knees, quadriceps, glutes
Sets: 3
Reps: 2–5 each leg
Rest: 30 seconds   **LEVEL 2**

The single-leg squat is a great exercise for strengthening the knee, but its major benefits here are improved control and stability of this joint; the exercise can also improve or maintain the knee ROM. It can be a challenging exercise for beginners, but we recommend starting with a shallow single-leg squat and focusing on balance and control at the knee; this will help protect and preserve the meniscus cartilages. In time, the increased squatting range will come, and with it, increased strength at the knee.

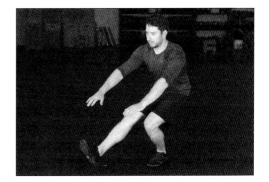

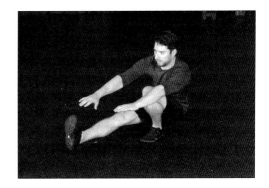

1. To perform the single-leg squat, stand on one foot with the other outstretched in front of you. Reach your arms forwards to aid with balance.
2. Bend your stance knee and start to squat down, keeping your stance foot flat on the floor. Aim to 'sit back' into the squat, ensuring that the knee does not pass forward of the toes.
3. As you descend, move your free foot forwards, straightening your knee as you do so.
4. Keep descending until you reach your current limit of ability; you may be able to descend so far that your posterior thigh touches your calf. This will be your end-point.
5. Pause for a second, and then use the quadriceps and glutes to push through the stance hip and knee until you are back at the starting position. This counts as one repetition. Repeat. Change legs.

Teaching Points

The single-leg squat can be very challenging. Start with a shallow squat, and if necessary use external support to help with control. We would recommend, however, trying to work without external support in order to develop your stability and control, and instead sacrificing the depth of the squat initially.

ITB Syndrome (Runner's Knee)

The ITB is a thick band of connective tissue called *fascia*; it runs from the outer upper thigh, travels down the outer thigh to cross the knee, and anchors into the outer upper shin (tibia). This fascial band has a crucial role in stabilising and supporting the knee during movement, but also provides a surface for attachment for some large muscles in the buttock, hip and thigh. With any repeated bending and straightening of the knee joint, especially under load (think of running and cycling), there is steady rubbing of the ITB over the lateral bony bump of the lower femur (Figure 9.7). This irritation leads to inflammation and pain, which can be experienced when moving off from rest.

ITB syndrome can be a particularly resistant and debilitating problem to have. As its other name suggests, this condition is common in runners, with whom it is the leading cause of lateral (outer) knee pain. The condition can also be experienced, however, with cycling, squatting and non-sporting populations.

Prevention is better than cure in this situation. Develop strong knees that are capable of moving regularly through a full range – Key Exercise 9.6 will help you get there! Avoid excessive load and repetitive knee movements until you have developed

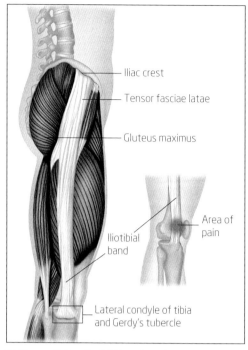

Labels:
- Iliac crest
- Tensor fasciae latae
- Gluteus maximus
- Iliotibial band
- Area of pain
- Lateral condyle of tibia and Gerdy's tubercle

■ **Figure 9.7.** Iliotibial band syndrome.

a strong base of strength and control. If you are currently experiencing ITB syndrome, manage the symptoms first before starting rehabilitation exercises. See a health or medical professional if you are stuck in the acute stage of runner's knee.

KEY EXERCISE 9.6: ITB FOAM ROLL

Target Area: ITB
Sets: 3
Duration: 30 seconds each leg
Rest: 30 seconds

LEVEL 1

The idea of stretching the ITB is controversial, so here we will discuss the mobility of this fibrous band and its associated structures. By exposing the ITB to foam rolling, you may be able to restore or improve its

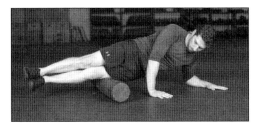

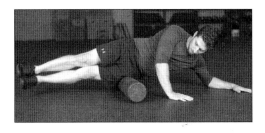

mobility relative to the structures around it. In consequence, the ITB may move over the outer knee more freely. Foam rolling can feel particularly painful in this region; we therefore suggest modifying the amount of body weight applied as your comfort dictates.

1. To perform the ITB foam roll, lie down on one side with the foam roller underneath your lower outer-thigh, at 90 degrees to your body.
2. Support your body weight with your hands, and then start to roll up and down the foam roller.
3. Keep your legs together and tense/brace them if it helps with stability. If there are any sore areas, spend more time and attention on these parts. You can also place the upper leg on the floor to support some of your body weight.
4. Roll for the required time, and then change legs and repeat.

Teaching Points

As with the other foam-rolling exercises, if you find that your legs are too sore to perform the movement properly, try using a softer foam roller. You can move on to a harder foam roller as your tolerance allows.

Also recommended: Key Exercise 8.5 (glute stretch), Exercise 9.10 (ITB mobilisation).

Bursitis

As we saw earlier in this chapter, there can be between 11 and 14 bursae in the average knee! Some are more susceptible to injury than others and this usually involves an excessive amount of friction or pressure at the site; the bursae will become swollen and painful in response. Bursae may also be injured through direct trauma, but that is not the focus of this book.

Commonly injured knee bursae include the prepatellar bursa, the infrapatellar bursa and the pes anserine ('goose-foot') bursa. Prepatellar bursitis is more commonly known as *housemaid's knee*, while infrapatellar bursitis is often named *clergyman's knee*; other causative professions have included *floor-layer's knee* and *plumber's knee*. Be careful, it is a dangerous world out there! We recommend avoiding the causative factors and using padding for kneeling activities. See a health or medical professional for advice on managing the acute symptoms of a knee bursitis. There are no specific body-weight exercises advised for this condition

KEY POINT *Prevention is better than cure for most injuries, including those to the knees. Develop strong knees that are capable of moving regularly through a full range.*

Knee Muscle and Tendon Problems

Niggling hamstring problems are the blight of many athletic individuals. These issues can prevent you from kicking a football, striding out during a run, or completing some lower-limb gym exercises. They can even niggle during day-to-day activities, such as bending forwards to pick something up or tying shoelaces. As a two-joint muscle, the hamstrings are susceptible to injury, and this is usually caused by a sudden stretch or rapid contraction. Over time, this injury may not settle fully and you can be left with a chronic hamstring strain. Subsequently, there will nearly always be muscle imbalances, with tightening and shortening of the hamstrings. Rehabilitate this fully, or better still prevent this type of injury, with Key Exercise 9.7.

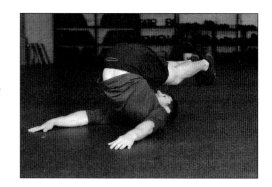

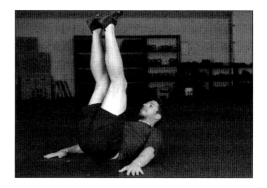

KEY EXERCISE 9.7: ROLLOVER INTO STRADDLE SIT

Target Area: Hamstrings, lower back, glutes, adductors
Sets: 3
Reps: 10
Rest: 30 seconds　　　　**LEVEL 2**

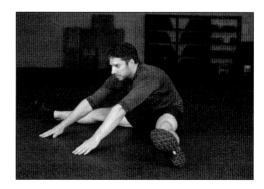

The rollover develops mobility and flexibility in the lower back, glutes and groin. The exercise is included here for its dynamic ability to stretch the hamstrings in two positions – first when the legs are overhead, and second when in the straddle sit (which can itself be done as a stand-alone exercise). Only take this movement as far as you are comfortable, and avoid excessive stress on the neck and head.

1. To perform the rollover into straddle sit, assume a seated position on the ground with your legs stretched out in front of you.

2. Now roll backwards onto your upper back and allow your straight legs to lower over your head. Place your hands by the sides of your head for increased support and stability.

3. Using a pushing action from your arms and also some work from your trunk, bring yourself forwards and upright to a seated position, but this time spread your legs into a wide straddle position. Once in this position, reach forwards between

your legs until you feel the stretch in the lower back and hamstrings. Hold this position for a second before repeating the exercise.

Teaching Points

The rollover part of this exercise requires trunk control and strength, making it an excellent bulletproof-body exercise by developing overall conditioning. If, however, you find this difficult, or you have a problem with your neck that precludes the rollover, just do the straddle sit stretch. This stretch will target the hamstrings, lower back and the adductor muscles (which also have a hamstring function!).

Also recommended: Key Exercise 8.3 (hamstring stretch), Exercise 9.8 (negative hamstring curl).

Following a history of overuse, the tendons of the hamstring muscles may become painful. Discomfort is usually experienced at the back of the knee and will be felt most when the knee flexes with resistance. The pain will be towards the outer or inner aspect of the posterior knee, and this will localise the problematic hamstring tendon. As we have seen in Chapters 5 and 6 of this book, tendon problems now tend to be regarded as *tendinopathies*, which means that rather than inflamed tendons they often show cellular signs of tendon breakdown. There is a sound body of evidence now to suggest that exercise therapy is a key part of rehabilitation for this problem. Progressive, loaded body-weight exercises may also defend against the development of tendinopathy. We offer Key Exercise 9.8 for this problem.

KEY EXERCISE 9.8: NEGATIVE HAMSTRING CURL

Target Area: Hamstrings, spinal extensor muscles
Sets: 3
Reps: 2–5
Rest: 30 seconds

LEVEL 3

Although performing hamstring curls on a machine is a great movement, the exercise can be modified to be even more effective with a bodyweight variation. The exercise presented here is in line with a well-evidenced rehabilitation program for hamstring problems, and will help you develop bulletproof thighs. The machine version of the hamstring curl is reversed by fixing the ankle and moving the body relative to the lower leg; this allows a body-weight exercise that activates the hips and trunk, which is an all-round win. There are many variations of this exercise, but we will focus on the negative version in order to develop the eccentric loading of the hamstring tendons and muscles. Note that it can be very difficult to find the specific piece of equipment required to perform the negative hamstring curl. If this is the case, you can perform the exercise with the aid of a partner, getting them to hold your ankles securely while you lower your torso towards the ground.

1. To perform the negative hamstring curl, start in the upright kneeling position. Secure your ankles and pad the underside of your knees.
2. Keeping the torso straight, begin to extend your knees and lower yourself towards the floor. Aim to make this movement slow

and controlled. Keep your hands out in front of you to guard against descending rapidly towards the floor.

3. Lower yourself as far as you feel able to. If this is not very far at first, do not worry – this will improve as your strength increases.

4. Return to the starting position. You can come out of the curl position by pushing yourself up with your arms (great for upper body strength), or by using your hamstrings to draw yourself back up.

5. Repeat.

Teaching Points

Variations on this exercise include the assisted and full hamstring curl (with eccentric and concentric phases). In the assisted version, you can use a stick/pole in your hands to push against the floor and support some of your upper body weight.

Also recommended: Key Exercise 8.3 (hamstring stretch), Key Exercise 9.7 (rollover to straddle sit).

Perhaps the most common tendon problem at the knee is patellar tendinopathy; again, this is not usually an inflamed tendon problem but a degenerative-type issue. The cause is usually excessive or unaccustomed load-bearing activity, which may be sports related (jumper's knee), but could equally be associated with an occupational activity. This type of problem can affect the tendon above or below the kneecap (patella), but most commonly affects the lower part of the tendon. A similar problem can affect the connective tissue 'expansions' on either side of the patella. Tendon failure and degeneration around the knee can lead to a gradual onset of pain around the front of the knee, and this may be worse with resisted knee extension. Tendinopathy problems appear to

respond well to gradually loaded exercise, in which body-weight exercises have a crucial role. Add Key Exercise 9.9 to your resilience or rehabilitation program, but be prepared to stick with it, since tendinopathies may take several weeks to respond to the load at a cellular level. If your pain worsens, we suggest you see a health or medical professional for tailored advice.

KEY EXERCISE 9.9: LUNGE

Target Area: Knees, quadriceps, patellar ligament
Sets: 3
Reps: 10 each leg
Rest: 30 seconds   **LEVEL 1**

The lunge is a great exercise for the knee, as each is loaded individually; this develops the added elements of stability and control. The exercise also imparts an eccentric (lengthening) load to the individual quadriceps and patellar ligament. You can also vary the difficulty, making it suitable for widely varying fitness and ability levels.

1. To perform the lunge, stand with your feet shoulder-width apart, arms by your sides in a relaxed posture.

2. Take a large step forwards with one leg, planting the foot firmly on the ground.

3. Bend the front knee and allow your rear knee to move towards the floor; this creates an eccentric load on the quadriceps and patellar ligament of the front knee.

4. Keep going until your front knee is bent at 90 degrees, and your rear knee is almost touching the ground. Now push up on the front leg to return to the starting position. Change legs and repeat.

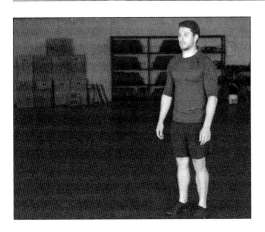

■ Body-weight Exercises for Improved Knee Function

EXERCISE 9.10: ITB MOBILISATION

Target Area: ITB, glutes, lateral quadriceps
Sets: 3
Duration: 20–30 seconds
Rest: 20 seconds

LEVEL 2

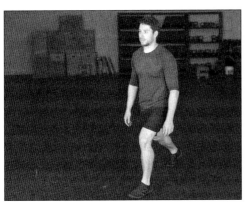

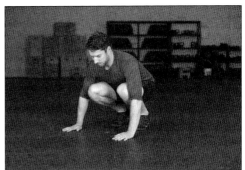

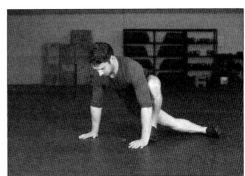

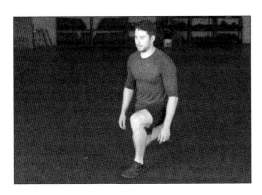

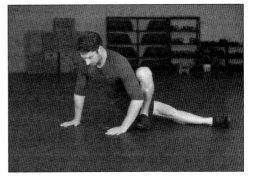

Teaching Points

If this exercise is too difficult, you can reduce the ROM to make it a lot easier. To do this, bend your knees by a smaller amount and only descend part way towards the ground. As you get stronger and more confident, you can keep descending all the way down to the floor.

The ITB provides a connective tissue anchor for some of the large muscles of the hip and thigh, and also stabilises the knee joint. Whether the ITB can be stretched is controversial, but the muscles that attach to it certainly can. The ITB 'mobilisation' suggested here is intended to improve mobility of the ITB in order to reduce the pressure where it crosses the outer knee.

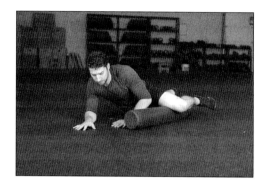

1. To perform the ITB mobilisation, crouch down with your hands and feet on the floor.
2. Move one leg sideways, making sure that it goes behind the leg that stays planted on the ground. Use your hands to support your body weight when you do this.
3. Keep stretching your leg out sideways, and rest this leg on the outside of your other foot. You should feel a strain in the outside of your leg, running from your hip down to your outer knee.
4. Hold this position for the required time, and then change legs and repeat.

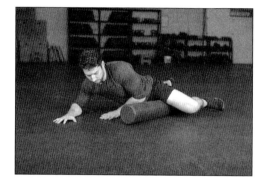

Teaching Points

The ITB mobilisation should help to alleviate any stress at the outer knee. If the injury is acute and the area is sore and inflamed, we recommend assessment and advice from a health or medical professional in the first instance.

On the opposite side to the abductor muscles and the ITB are the adductor muscles. These muscles act to bring the leg in towards the centre line of the body, and also help in stabilisation of the hip and knee during running, jumping, squatting and other lower body movements. Foam rolling this area can help to improve any soft-tissue restrictions.

EXERCISE 9.11: ADDUCTOR FOAM ROLL

Target Area: Adductor muscles of the thigh
Sets: 3
Duration: 30 seconds each leg
Rest: 20 seconds

LEVEL 2

1. To perform the adductor foam roll, position your foam roller parallel to your torso, and crouch down on top of it.
2. Keep one leg straight and bend the other at the knee, placing the inside of your thigh on top of the foam roller.
3. Support yourself on your hands, and start to roll backwards and forwards over the roller. Work all the way up to the groin area, and then down to the top of the knee.
4. Keep rolling for 30 seconds, and then change legs and repeat.

Teaching Points

As with the other foam-rolling exercises, you will want to start with a softer foam roller or reduce your body-weight pressure against the roller.

■ Goal Exercises for the Knee

Goal exercises have been presented in other chapters of this book both to serve as a measure of your general body-weight strength and fitness, and to provide you with developmental exercises that can be incorporated in a bulletproof-body exercise routine. The knee joint is no exception – a few exercises for developing lower-limb strength and injury resistance are given below. Combine these with the goal exercises in Chapters 8 and 10 for a fuller workout.

GOAL EXERCISE 9.12: ICE SKATER

Target Area: Knees, quadriceps
Sets: 3
Reps: 10 (5 each leg)
Rest: 30 seconds   **LEVEL 2**

The ice skater will test the strength of the lower body as well as promote good stability in the knees. This exercise requires adequate jumping ability; therefore, if you have knee or lower body joint problems, seek advice from your medical professional beforehand. The ice skater can be thought of as a natural progression from the lunge (Exercise 9.10). Ideally, wear shoes with good grip and use a non-slip floor surface.

1. To perform the ice skater, stand in a neutral position and keep the arms relaxed.

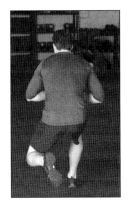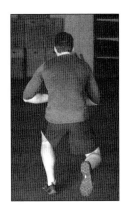

2. From here, move your weight onto one foot and jump forwards at an angle, aiming to land with the opposite foot.
3. As you land on one foot, bend the knee to absorb the shock.
4. Jump forwards again at an angle, but this time to the other side, and land on the opposite foot. Keep doing this for the required repetitions (or distance if preferred), and then rest.

Teaching Points

The multidirectional and dynamic stress of this exercise contribute to improved knee stability. The further you jump both forwards and laterally, the greater the stress put on the knees. If you are just starting out with this exercise, begin by making small jumps, gradually moving up in difficulty as your strength and mobility progress.

GOAL EXERCISE 9.13: JUMP SQUAT

Target Area: Knees, quadriceps, glutes, calves
Sets: 3
Reps: 15 (or 20 seconds duration)
Rest: 45 seconds   **LEVEL 3**

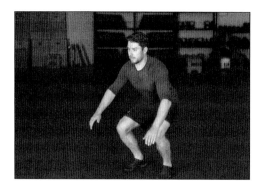

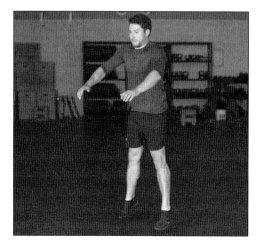

In this exercise we introduce an explosive component to the mix. The squat is great for the hips and knees in general, but the jump squat adds an element of instability to the movement, especially on the landing phase. The forces applied to the knees are also higher because of the deceleration required to counteract the downward movement. Before attempting this exercise, make sure that you are fully versed and experienced in the normal body-weight squat (Key Exercise 9.1) and the deep squat position (Key Exercise 8.2).

1. To perform the jump squat, stand with your feet shoulder-width apart, toes pointing out slightly, and your arms loose by your sides.

2. Squat down, bending the knees, pushing the hips back and down, and moving the arms forwards to aid balance.
3. Keep descending until your thighs are parallel to the ground. If you really want to push the boundaries, continue until you reach the deep squat position.
4. Push up hard, extending your hips, knees and ankles as forcefully as possible. Jump into the air, keeping your eyes looking forwards to stay balanced.
5. Land under control, immediately bending the knees, descending into the squat position once again. Continue for the desired number of reps, or for a set period of time.

Teaching Points

As with any explosive or plyometric exercise, care must be taken not to subject the target area to excessive force. If you are working with the jump squat for the first time, or have had some time away from training and are returning to it, start small and build up. Do this by only descending until your thighs are horizontal and only jumping into the air a few centimetres. As time progresses and you become stronger and more confident, you can descend lower and jump higher.

GOAL EXERCISE 9.14: JUMP LUNGE

Target Area: Knees, quadriceps
Sets: 3
Reps: 10 (or 20 seconds duration)
Rest: 45 seconds

LEVEL 3

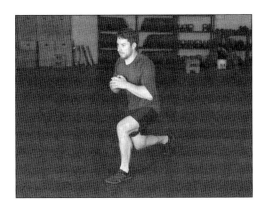

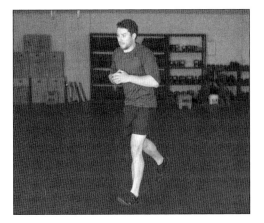

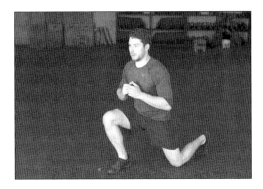

In addition to the jump squat there is the jump lunge. This is the same type of progression from the lunge as the jump squat from the body-weight squat. The instability and coordination required in the jump lunge, however, is higher than in both squat

variations. Each knee will be tested vigorously, and each repetition will require the positions of the feet to be swapped in mid-air; this introduces a coordination requirement that may come easily (or not), depending on your training experience. We recommend only attempting this when you are comfortable with the jump squat.

1. To perform the jump lunge, stand in a stretched-out lunge position, with both knees nearly straight. Let your arms hang loosely by your sides, ready to help with balance.
2. From here, descend to the floor, bending both knees by an equal amount so that your torso stays vertical. Stop just short of your rear knee touching the ground.
3. Push up hard, extending your hips, knees and ankles and jumping into the air.
4. Once you are in the air, move your front leg backwards and your rear leg forwards. You should be aiming to land with your feet the same distance apart as when you started.
5. Land under control, bending both knees to absorb the shock. Descend to the bottom position immediately, to prepare for the next repetition.

Teaching Points

The jump lunge is a demanding exercise, but it can be made easier by simply reducing the ROM and the intensity of the movement. You can accomplish this by not dropping as low when descending towards the floor, and by not jumping as high when leaving the ground. As you get stronger and more confident, you can start to descend all the way and jump as high into the air as possible.

10

The Lower Leg, Ankle and Foot

■ **Introduction to the Lower Leg, Ankle and Foot**

Humans have been walking on two legs for about two million years, with evidence of bipedal locomotion (walking on two legs) in primates extending back four million years. Over this period of time, the foot and ankle have evolved, with the development of enlarged heels for weight bearing, smaller toes for supporting rather than grasping, and arched rather than flat feet. The result is a platform to support the entire weight of the body, and a mechanism for transferring that weight in an energy-efficient way. Despite the fact that human walking is 75% more efficient than human running, we have managed amazing feats of athletic ability, from running the marathon in 2 hours 3 minutes to sprinting 100m in 9.58 seconds.

As babies, we must learn this most fundamental of human skills, which can take on average 12–15 months to master. Along the way, there are trips and falls as our ability to maintain balance over two feet is constantly challenged. In this chapter we look at some of the key locomotive structures of the lower leg, ankle and foot that keep us up and running. We will also explore some common injuries and dysfunction of this region, and finish with a range of body-weight exercises to keep you on your toes!

■ **Functional Anatomy of the Lower Leg, Ankle and Foot**

Passive Structures

As we saw in Chapter 9, the tibia is a large weight-bearing bone of the lower limb and forms part of the knee joint. The tibia transmits the weight of the upper body and thigh and transfers it to the talus bone in the ankle joint. Alongside the heavy-duty tibia sits the more slender fibula bone. The distance between these two bones is spanned along their length by a fibrous membrane, creating a firm union between the bones but allowing a certain degree of flexing when weight bearing; this flexing ability of the fibula and the joining membrane is put to the test when landing on the feet from a height. The end of the fibula is slightly lower than the tibia, with both of these long bones having endings that create a mortise for the talus bone to sit in. The bony structure of the lower leg and ankle is shown in Figure 10.1.

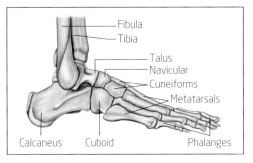

■ **Figure 10.1.**   The bony structures of the foot and ankle joint, lateral view.

The talus bone of the ankle sits on the heel bone (calcaneus) and transfers the body weight to the ground through the heel and the rest of the foot. The foot is made up of 26 bones that form a total of 33 intricate joints. All of these joints, including those of the ankle, are supported by ligaments that bind the bones together and prevent unwanted movements. The ligaments on the outer side of the ankle can be stressed during an ankle sprain, as we shall see later in this chapter. The bones of the foot form a natural arch, and this contributes to the spring in our step; this bony architecture can be seen in Figure 10.1. In addition to the numerous ligaments of the foot and ankle, the load-bearing ability of the foot is increased by a connective tissue structure called the *plantar fascia*: this tough fibrous band sits under the length of the foot and supports the arch.

Active Structures

The lower leg houses the powerful calf muscle known as the *gastrocnemius*: this muscle is capable of pulling on the heel bone (calcaneus) via the strong Achilles tendon to raise you up on tip-toes, allowing you to walk and run. Several other muscles can be found in the lower leg; these contribute to postural stability and control, keeping you upright against gravity for up to several hours at a time when standing. The numerous tendons of these muscles, shown in Figure 10.2, cross the ankle joint and contribute to the dynamic stability and movement of this joint.

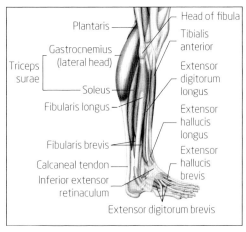

■ **Figure 10.2.**   The muscles and tendons of the lower leg and ankle, lateral view.

The muscles at the front of the shin cross the ankle and contract to draw your foot and toes towards your shin in a movement called *dorsiflexion*. A key muscle here is the tibialis anterior, which is hard at work when you walk on your heels. The fibularis brevis and longus muscles run down the outside of the lower leg and ankle, and pull on the foot when you turn the soles of your feet outwards. This muscle activity contributes to maintaining and supporting the arches of the foot, and is also important in protecting the outer ankle from 'inversion' ankle sprains.

> **KEY POINT**   *Muscles in the lower leg provide powerful propulsive forces, have incredible endurance in maintaining balance during standing, support the arches of the feet, and contribute to the stability of the ankle joint.*

■ Common Lower Leg, Ankle and Foot Dysfunction

Calf Strain

Excessive or sudden loading of the calf muscles can lead to tearing of some of the fibres in the muscles at the back of the lower leg. If only a few fibres are affected, you may notice little impact on your daily or sporting activities other than some muscle soreness. The greater the number of disrupted fibres, the more pronounced the pain and limitation. If the calf injury is acute and you are uncertain about the degree of damage, we recommend that you seek assessment by a qualified health or medical professional.

Tennis leg is a type of calf strain that can affect the plantaris (a deep muscle of the calf) or commonly the powerful gastrocnemius muscle. Gastrocnemius has two sections or 'heads' to it; the inner (medial) head is the one more prone to tear or partially rupture. If you have been advised to exercise for rehabilitation of a calf strain, or have a recurrent injury in this region, add Key Exercise 10.1 to your training program to build resilience in this muscle group.

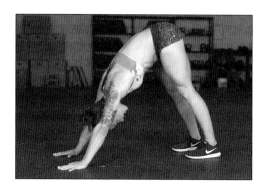

any other. The downward dog uses multiple joints and muscles simultaneously, and is the ultimate definition of a body-weight exercise. We include it here for its benefits in developing length under tension at the calf, but also for mobilising the ankle, mobilising the sciatic nerve and stretching the hamstrings. Dysfunction in any of these areas can contribute to ongoing calf problems.

1. To perform the downward dog, assume a push-up position and walk your feet towards your hands while keeping your knees straight. Walk in as far as you can until you have taken up the strain across the back of the legs, the lower back and the shoulders.
2. Keep your feet facing forwards and try to place your heels flat on the ground. Ensure that you have safely loaded your arms and shoulders by spreading the fingers wide, with the middle finger facing forwards and the palms shoulder-width apart.
3. Use straight elbows to support your weight, but do not lock them out. Push backwards through the arms to adjust the strain in the calf muscles.
4. With the feet hip-width apart, press the heels into the floor to create a stretch in the back of the legs. Try a slight bend in the knees if you need to focus the stretch on the calves.
5. Keep the back flat and relax the neck. Hold the position for 20 seconds.

KEY EXERCISE 10.1: DOWNWARD DOG

Target Area: Ankle joints, calf muscles, sciatic nerve, wrists, shoulders, spine
Sets: 3
Duration: Hold for 20–30 seconds
Rest: 30 seconds　　　**LEVEL 2**

Yoga fans will be no strangers to this exercise and will quickly tell you about its benefits. If you have never done yoga before, we recommend that you try this exercise over

Teaching Points

This is a true bulletproof-body exercise that develops strength, stamina and suppleness in multiple body areas. If you have weakness or pain in any other region of your body while doing this exercise, we recommend that you address those issues first by consulting other chapters of this book. Do not perform this exercise if you have uncontrolled high blood pressure.

Ankle Sprain

Sprains of the outer ankle ligaments are the most common ankle injury and usually involve an 'inversion' injury, whereby you roll over the outside of your ankle (Figure 10.3). Lateral ankle sprains are graded according to severity, from a mild overstretch (grade 1) to a complete rupture (grade 3). Most people, however, will experience a partial ligament tear (grade 2), but if you are unsure, first seek the attention of a health or medical professional. A *chronic lateral ankle sprain* is one that has a history of spraining and

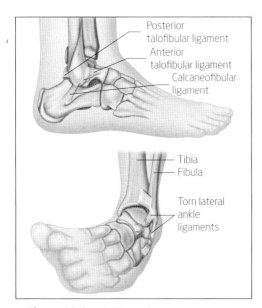

■ **Figure 10.3.** Ankle sprain.

never fully settles, or keeps recurring. There may be instability, pain or ongoing swelling/inflammation. Functional rehabilitation of the ankle is the goal here, and this should include proprioceptive retraining (see below), and the development of muscular stability and control at the ankle joint. Rehabilitation should be continued for anything up to several months to fully regain lost function at the ankle. Key Exercise 10.2 is an essential part of an ankle sprain rehabilitation program.

KEY EXERCISE 10.2: SINGLE-LEG BALANCE

Target Area: Ankles
Sets: 3
Duration: Hold for 20–60 seconds
Rest: 30 seconds   LEVEL 1

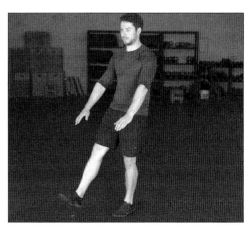

You might think that body-weight exercises do not come any simpler than this, but they also do not come any more effective in terms of regaining ankle function. *Proprioception* is the body's internal sense of the relative position of body parts and their efforts during movement. Put more simply, it is the ability of a joint (here, your ankle) to respond quickly and subconsciously to stresses placed on it. This straightforward exercise helps retrain this function and creates a base for developing more complex exercises.

1. To perform the single-leg balance, assume a standing position on a firm, non-slip surface. Slowly place increasing body weight onto the affected ankle until you are standing on one leg. The aim is to challenge balance, so where possible do not hold onto anything, but have a stable support close by should you lose balance.
2. You may begin to wobble slightly during the exercise, but do not worry, as this is the point. If you occasionally need to touch down with the other foot, that is allowable too.
3. Hold for the required time and really focus on maintaining your balance, even if you sway a lot. Change legs to compare the ability of each side.

Teaching Points

If this exercise is too easy, you can progress it in several ways. Try standing on a more challenging surface, try with your eyes closed, have someone throw a ball to you to catch, or juggle a ball while standing on the one leg. All of these will further challenge your balance ability. As you make progress, add sport-specific movements or plyometric jumps and maintain your balance on landing.

Achilles Tendon Dysfunction

The Achilles tendon is the longest tendon in the body and is thought to have a tensile strength capable of withstanding forces of up to 12 times body weight. It is a common site for injury and is susceptible to tears and even complete rupture. More likely, though, is the development of a *tendinopathy*, a degenerative change within the tendon that leads to pain, tendon thickening and stiffness. The onset of this problem is usually gradual, and the pain can persist for many months. Excessive or unaccustomed forces through the Achilles tendon are the likely cause of tendinopathy; the problem is commonly seen in athletic populations of all levels, and generally between the mid-thirties and the early fifties. To determine whether your Achilles pain is due to tendinopathy or a tear, we recommend you seek assessment from a qualified health or medical professional.

Management of Achilles tendon pain caused by degenerative change should include a modification of the causative factor. Return to sport may take up to three months as the tendon adapts to a progressive load. This load can be applied through body-weight exercise very effectively, and the use of eccentric loading in the calf muscles has gained popularity as an effective treatment. Key Exercise 10.3 shows you how to apply an eccentric load through the Achilles tendon.

KEY EXERCISE 10.3: NEGATIVE CALF RAISE

Target Area: Ankle joints, calf muscles
Sets: 3
Reps: 10–20
Rest: 30 seconds

LEVEL 1

The muscles of the calf are responsible for much of the strength necessary for ankle plantar flexion, an essential requirement for

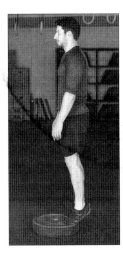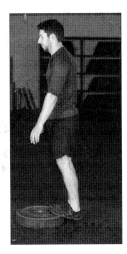

walking, running and jumping activities. Make yourself more resilient to calf injury, and possibly increase athletic performance, by working on this exercise. The negative calf raise uses body weight effectively to build strength and also to develop ankle mobility.

1. To perform the negative calf raise, stand on a step or platform with your toes on the edge. Hold onto something to aid your balance.
2. Use your calf muscles to raise your heels as high as possible. Think about pointing your toes to make this happen. This is the starting position.
3. Allow your heels to lower slowly to create an eccentric (lengthening) contraction of the calf muscles. Keep lowering until you feel a stretch in the these muscles. Hold this position for a second, before quickly contracting the calf muscles to return to the starting position. This counts as one repetition.
4. Repeat.

Teaching Points

If you find that just using your own body weight is not enough resistance, you can add weight to this movement. The easiest way to do this is to perform the exercise while standing on one leg. Once you have done the required number of repetitions, change legs. Alternatively, hold a dumbbell in each hand; start with a light weight, and build up from there.

Plantar Fasciitis

The plantar fascia is a strong connective tissue structure that runs under the length of the foot and contributes to the load-bearing function of the foot by supporting the arches. The plantar fascia anchors to the underside of the heel bone (calcaneus), and this is a potential site of injury and pain. Pain in the heel may be due to plantar fasciitis, usually resulting from small tears in the fascia through microtrauma or traction stress. Whether heel spurs are relevant in this pain condition is debatable, since these calcium deposits have been found in people not experiencing heel pain.

Whether the plantar fascia can be stretched is questionable, although it is acknowledged there is probably some 'give' in the structure when under load. Despite this uncertainty, there exists some research to suggest that stretching the plantar fascia may be an effective treatment. If you have this condition, you could also consider reviewing your choice of footwear, modifying any aggravating activity, and developing the small muscles of the feet through exercise and load bearing. Key Exercise 10.4 is a good place to start.

KEY EXERCISE 10.4: MODIFIED FROG STANCE

Target Area: Ankle joints, plantar fasciae
Sets: 3
Duration: Hold for 10–20 seconds, once in position
Rest: 30 seconds

LEVEL 2

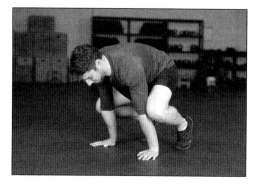

The modified frog stance is a variation of the frog stance (Key Exercise 5.2) – a gold-standard body-weight exercise seen in Chapter 5. This is a testament to body-weight exercises that incorporate multiple joints and soft tissues – you get an all-over workout in one go!

In this modification the key is to focus on the ankle and toe positions, aiming to flex (dorsiflex) the foot and toes simultaneously. Use the support of the arms to control the stretch through the foot and therefore the plantar fascia.

1. To perform the modified frog stance, place your hands on the floor in front of you, with your fingers facing forwards or slightly outwards and your hands shoulder-width apart.
2. Position your knees on the outsides of your elbows, as far forwards as you can

manage. If flexibility at the hips is an issue, refer to Chapter 8 of this book, but just do what you can for now.

3. Lean forwards onto your hands and onto the balls of your feet. In this position your ankles and toes will be flexed and this should be felt as a stretch through the plantar fascia. If you need to take some of this load off the plantar fascia, continue to lean forwards and place more load onto the arms. Leaning forwards can also be used to add further stretch by further flexing the toes; however, do not lean so far forwards that your feet leave the ground (unless you want to add a shoulder and hip workout at the same time!).

Teaching Points

Use the arms to add or reduce loading on the plantar fascia. You may find that the initial starting position is sufficient. When you are comfortable in this position you can slowly roll backwards and forwards on the balls of your feet to mobilise the plantar fascia.

Osteoarthritis of the Ankle

The ankle is not a common site for osteoarthritis, but you may have a history of ankle injury, fracture or excessive occupational or sporting use. *Osteoarthritis* is a degenerative condition of the cartilage on the surfaces of joining bones, and is associated with risk factors including obesity, being over 40 years of age, and biomechanical changes to the joint (resulting from, for example, flat feet or unsuitable footwear).

If you have a degree of osteoarthritis in the ankle joint, you may find that you have slightly more limitation when pointing your toes away from you (plantar flexion) than when drawing your toes towards you (dorsiflexion). Work gradually into Key Exercise 10.5 to restore some of this movement and ease any joint stiffness.

KEY EXERCISE 10.5: HEEL SIT

Target Area: Ankle joints, muscles at the front of the shins
Sets: 3
Duration: Hold for 10–20 seconds
Rest: 30 seconds

LEVEL 2

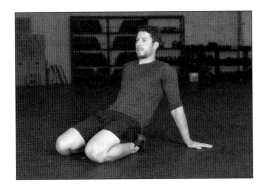

The heel sit exercise uses body weight to stretch the front of the ankle joints while also flexing the knees. Do not hold this position for too long, as you may place excessive strain on the knees and ankles. Use the time while in this position to do some breathing exercises, and even practise some relaxation or mindfulness. Just remember to cushion your knees first on a comfortable surface.

1. To perform the heel sit, take up a kneeling position on a comfortable surface. Place your feet behind you with the ankles in a plantar-flexed position.
2. Sit back onto your heels and take up as much strain on the fronts of the ankles as is comfortable. Use your body weight to add load. Hold for the required time.

3. Come slowly out of the stretch into a high kneeling position. Rest for a moment in this position, before sitting back onto the heels and repeating the stretch.

Teaching Points

This simple exercise can improve joint mobility and function of the ankles. It is also a great stretch for the muscles at the front of the shins and may be used where there is compartment syndrome present.

■ **Body-weight Exercises for Improved Lower Leg, Ankle and Foot Function**

EXERCISE 10.6: UNLOADED DORSIFLEXION

Target Area: Ankle joints, calf muscles
Sets: 3
Reps: 10 each leg
Rest: 20 seconds

LEVEL 1

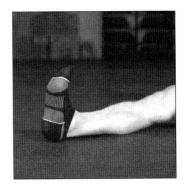

As the ankles can be elevated relatively easily, we can use this position to perform unloaded (without weight) ankle mobility exercises. There are four of these exercises, corresponding to the four movements that occur naturally around the ankle.

The first of these exercises, unloaded dorsiflexion, can be used to increase or maintain ROM, to gently load recovering soft-tissue after injury or to aide circulation.

1. To perform unloaded dorsiflexion, sit or lie down, making sure that the ankle is supported but free to move.
2. From here, use your lower leg muscles to pull your foot towards your shin. Curl your toes up as well, to help increase the ROM.
3. Hold this position for a second or so, and then relax your ankle. Perform the required number of repetitions. Change legs and repeat.

The unloaded ankle plantar-flexion exercise increases mobility at the ankle joint, but also primes the calf muscles for more vigorous body-weight exercise. It is also good for maintaining circulation in the leg if you are immobilised for any reason. *Plantar flexion* describes the downward movement of the foot or, more simply, pointing of the toes. Focus on this position when performing this exercise.

1. To perform unloaded plantar flexion, sit or lie down, making sure that the ankle is supported but free to move.
2. Use your lower leg muscles to point your toes. Scrunch your toes towards the sole of your foot to help increase the ROM.
3. Hold this position for a second or so, and then relax your ankle. Perform the required number of repetitions. Change legs and repeat.

EXERCISE 10.7: UNLOADED PLANTAR FLEXION

Target Area: Ankle joints, anterior tibial muscles
Sets: 3
Reps: 10 each leg
Rest: 20 seconds   **LEVEL 1**

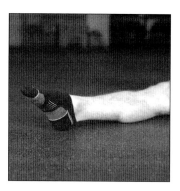

EXERCISE 10.8: UNLOADED INVERSION

Target Area: Ankle joints, lateral ankle ligaments
Sets: 3
Reps: 10 each leg
Rest: 20 seconds   **LEVEL 1**

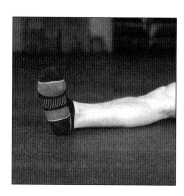

The unloaded ankle inversion exercise is very useful for mobilising the ankle joint, but also for developing a therapeutic stress on the outer ankle ligaments after an ankle sprain. Performing this exercise in an unloaded position reduces the risk of further injury in the early stages of rehabilitation.

1. To perform unloaded inversion, sit or lie down, making sure that the ankle is supported but free to move.
2. Use your lower leg muscles to pull your foot inwards so that the sole of your foot points towards your other foot. For comparison purposes, do the exercise on both ankles simultaneously.
3. Hold this position for a second or so, and then relax your ankle. Perform the required number of repetitions. Change legs if doing the exercise one ankle at a time, and repeat.

1. To perform unloaded eversion, sit or lie down, making sure that the ankle is supported but free to move.
2. From here, use your lower leg muscles to pull your foot outwards so that the sole of your foot points away from your other foot.
3. Hold for a second or so, and then relax your ankle. Perform the required number of repetitions. Change legs and repeat.

EXERCISE 10.10: ANTERIOR TIBIAL MUSCLE STRETCH

Target Area: Quadriceps, anterior tibial muscles
Sets: 3
Duration: 20–30 seconds
Rest: 20 seconds

`LEVEL 1`

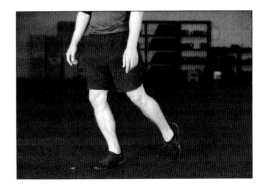

EXERCISE 10.9: UNLOADED EVERSION

Target Area: Ankle joints, fibularis muscles
Sets: 3
Reps: 10 each leg
Rest: 20 seconds

`LEVEL 1`

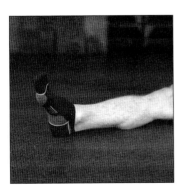

The muscles in front of the shin, including the tibialis anterior, can come under strain with repeated running, cycling and jumping activities. Pain can start after an activity level or type not previously done, and also when running in footwear that is too tight or too loose, or otherwise does not fit properly. The painful condition experienced may be a type of 'shin splints'. Try this stretch along with Key Exercise 10.5 to help keep this area flexible and functioning properly.

1. To perform the anterior tibial muscle stretch, stand up straight, with one foot flat on the ground and the other supported on the toes.
2. Pull the heel towards your buttocks by bending at the knee and holding the foot in a plantar-flexed position as shown in the image, so that you feel the stretch in the front of the shin. Keep the thighs parallel and push forwards at the hip to increase the stretch.
3. To add mobility at the ankle, you may want to rotate your ankle around slowly. Hold this position for 20–30 seconds. Change legs and repeat.

EXERCISE 10.11: CALF STRETCH

Primary Target Area: Ankle and calf muscles
Sets: 3
Duration: Hold for 20–30 seconds
Rest: 20 seconds

LEVEL 1

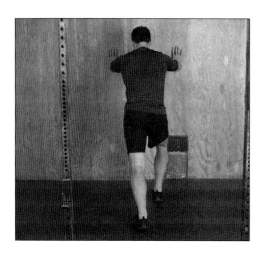

Stretching the calves is good practice for maintaining full ROM at the ankle and the knee, as the gastrocnemius muscle crosses both of these joints. The calf stretch also maintains the tone and length of the calf muscles and regularly loads the Achilles tendon. There are many ways to perform the stretch, but we have found that the following method is a practical approach to achieving the above aims, and can be adjusted to suit varying levels of flexibility.

1. To perform the calf stretch, stand facing a wall. Position the toes of one foot against the wall and the other foot approximately 60cm (24″) behind you. The feet should be pointing forwards.
2. Keeping the heel of your rear foot against the ground, lean forwards into the wall, supporting your weight with your arms. You should feel a stretch in the bottom of your rear leg; if not, move your rear foot further away from the wall.
3. Hold this position for 20–30 seconds, and then switch legs and repeat.

Teaching Points

If you find that the method outlined above does not provide sufficient stretch, you can perform it in the following way. Stand on the edge of a step or stair, with the toes of both feet just in contact with the platform. From this position, allow your heels to drop towards the ground. Keep lowering the heels until you reach the limit of your stretch, hold for the required amount of time and then rest.

■ Goal Exercises for the Lower Leg, Ankle and Foot

Goal exercises are suggested here for further developing the rehabilitation and resilience of the lower leg and ankle. These particular exercises can be added to your training program to build strength and mobility, and also act as a test of your physical condition.

GOAL EXERCISE 10.12: SKIPPING

Target Area: Calf muscles, ankles, cardiovascular fitness
Sets: 3
Duration: 30–60 seconds
Rest: 45–60 seconds

LEVEL 2

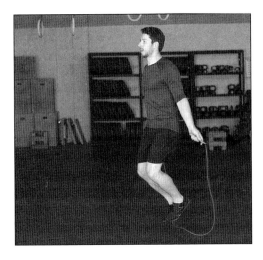

There is no better exercise for working your calves and keeping you on your toes than skipping with a rope. If you take this exercise up for this first time, be warned that you will feel it in the calf muscles, so go easy at first. It is a classic exercise for boxers to get them bouncing on their toes and also to develop cardiovascular fitness.

1. With or without a skipping rope, start gently by bouncing on the balls of your feet, either transferring your weight from one foot to the other or distributing your weight evenly on both feet at the same time.
2. Once the calf muscles are warm, increase the depth of the bounce, again shifting your weight or maintaining equal load on the feet.
3. Now add in a few high jumps, tucking your knees towards your chest. Settle back into a bounce while you get your breath back. Repeat the high jumps when ready.

Teaching Points

When you get fitter and more confident, you can mix things up with single-leg skipping, doubling up the jumps per rope swing, or even crossing the rope. You will have calves like Rocky Balboa in no time with this body-weight winner!

11
The Spine

■ Introduction to the Spine

In this chapter we will explore the wondrous
structure that is the spine. Although the
spine is one continuous integral structure
(Figure 11.1), it can be broken down from
a movement and support perspective into
three main sections:

• Cervical spine (neck)
• Thoracic spine (upper back)
• Lumbar spine (lower back)

When considering the global effects and
benefits of body-weight exercise, it is difficult
to say very much about the impact on neck
problems, other than the benefits that come
from improved neck and shoulder posture.
Improving thoracic spine and shoulder
posture can translate into significant
reductions in general neck pain. This pain
reduction occurs because the thoracic spine is
the base on which the cervical spine sits, and
having a slumped chest, ribcage and shoulders
will lead to poor neck posture. Postural
changes in the neck place the muscles,
ligaments, joints and discs of the cervical
spine under additional loads, thus leading

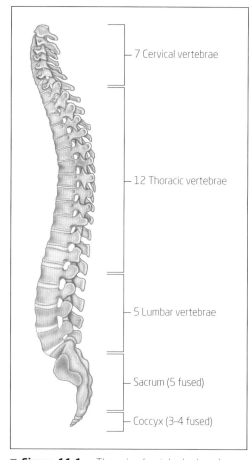

7 Cervical vertebrae

12 Thoracic vertebrae

5 Lumbar vertebrae

Sacrum (5 fused)

Coccyx (3-4 fused)

■ **Figure 11.1.** The spine (vertebral column),
lateral view.

to pain and dysfunction. Accordingly, the cervical spine section below will give a brief overview of the need-to-know anatomy of the neck to help you understand and appreciate the role of good posture. A key exercise to aid in addressing postural dysfunction of the neck will also be offered in due course.

Should your neck pain persist, or if you develop arm pain or symptoms such as pins and needles, reduced arm power or changes in sensation, you are advised to seek qualified and experienced assessment. You may find in this instance that strenuous activity of any type aggravates your neck pain, and so it would be unwise to persist with body-weight exercises in general.

The thoracic and lumbar spines can be a common source of pain that can limit daily function; this could include problems such as twisting to reach for a seatbelt, bending to put on shoes and socks, and of course limitation of sport and exercise pursuits. These two spinal regions will also be given consideration here and will be outlined in relation to body-weight exercises to condition and rehabilitate this most crucial of body structures.

◾ Functional Anatomy of the Spine

Cervical Spine

The neck is formed by the cervical spine, a critical structure that supports and moves the head. It houses the blood vessels and nervous tissue that connect the brain with the rest of the body, and is thus a vulnerable region. We would therefore not recommend loaded body-weight exercises here unless they are performed under the direction of a suitably qualified health or fitness professional.

Seven vertebral bones make up the cervical spine, with discs cushioning the spaces between them from the second to the seventh vertebrae and beyond. The cervical spine is built for mobility, with much of this movement coming from small facet joints on either side of adjacent vertebrae. In addition to the discs and the vertebral bones and their joints, the neck has multiple ligaments that reinforce the structures and their movements. The relationship of adjacent vertebrae and all of their shared structures is commonly referred to as a *motion segment*. An outline of the cervical spine structure can be seen in Figure 11.2.

The underlying shape of the vertebral bones and the discs gives the neck a natural forward curvature; this is termed a *lordosis*.

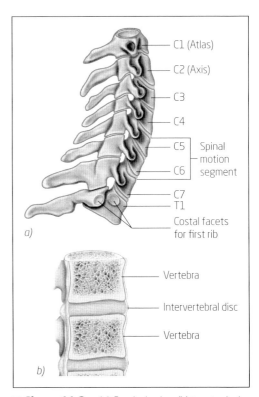

■ **Figure 11.2.** (a) Cervical spine; (b) two typical vertebrae and intervertebral disc.

The degree of postural lordosis differs in all of us; however, given the modern lifestyles that many of us have, the cervical lordosis is likely to be an exaggerated one. Poor sitting postures and prolonged use of electronic screens, such as smartphones and laptops, can contribute to this. If you look at the motion segment illustrated in Figure 11.2, you may begin to appreciate the load that this increased postural lordosis places on the discs, facet joints and ligaments. To offload the stress of postural neck pain, we offer a key exercise in the common spinal dysfunction section below; this exercise will also stretch the short and tight muscles at the back of the neck, which may be giving you neck and head pain.

Each motion segment of the spine is acted upon by multiple muscles to create a complex pattern of movements. The movement of rotation mostly comes from the upper part of the neck, between the first and second cervical vertebrae (C1 and C2), while the movements of flexion, extension and side flexion come from the lower cervical section (C3 to C7). Some examples of the muscles acting on the neck are outlined in Figure 11.3.

As can be seen in Figure 11.3, there are many muscles in the neck region, and most of them have tricky names! There are also other muscles to be aware of, such as the trapezius muscles, but the great news is that you do not need to know about individual muscles. It is believed that the brain works in terms of movement patterns, not individual muscle recruitment; good-quality movements will therefore condition the muscles of the neck for normal functioning.

> **KEY POINT** *The brain works in movement patterns, not individual muscle recruitment. Good-quality movements will condition the muscles of the neck for normal functioning.*

A final comment on neck anatomy should include a consideration of the nerve roots. These neural structures emerge at each level of the spine from above the first cervical vertebra (C1) to beyond the lowest level of the lumbar spine (L5), as we shall see later. There are eight nerve roots leaving either side of the cervical spine, as can be seen in Figure 11.4, and irritation or impingement of these structures can give you symptoms in the head, neck, shoulder, arm or hand.

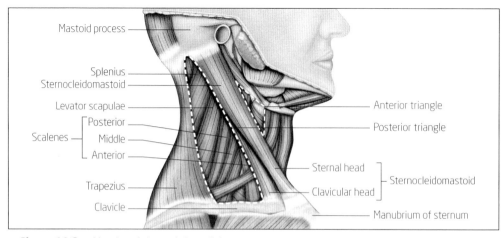

■ **Figure 11.3.** Muscles of the neck, lateral view.

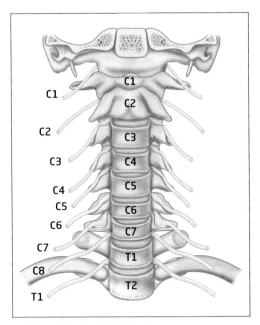

■ **Figure 11.4.** Cervical spine nerve roots.

A suitably qualified health or medical professional should assess such symptoms before you start any physical activity, including body-weight exercise. You may find, however, that simple ROM exercises (for example, Key Exercise 11.2) may ease some of your symptoms. Our advice would be to maintain these movements within your pain-free range.

Thoracic Spine

Compared with the spinal regions lying above and below it, the thoracic spine is a relatively stiff area. The ribcage contributes to this immobility by fixing most of the thoracic spine to the breast bone (sternum) at the front of the chest. The major benefit of this is that the internal organs of the heart and lungs are protected in a bony cage. There is, however, a certain amount flexing in this spinal region, as you will notice when you breathe in and out. It is this small degree of movement, and the structures that facilitate it, that can come under strain and generate pain.

The basic structure of the thoracic spine (Figure 11.5) follows the same blueprint that gave us the cervical spine outlined earlier. Twelve thicker vertebral bones are

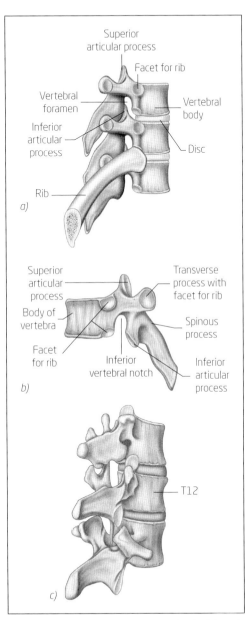

■ **Figure 11.5.** (a) Thoracic spine; b) typical thoracic vertebra [T6]; (c) the change in angle between the facet joints lends itself to the movements that are possible at each section of vertebrae.

all cushioned by discs that transmit an increasing load from structures above; the discs also act to stabilise this section of the spine. The combination of these structures, along with the ligaments and rib attachments, means that the thoracic spine has limited movement. That said, the facet joints of the thoracic spine are angled to allow greater rotation than the lumbar spine, while still allowing some forward flexion, side flexion and extension. In the space created in front of the thoracic facet joints, the pairs of nerve roots leave at each level from below T1 to T12. Symptoms from these structures are thought to be relatively rare.

Unlike the cervical and lumbar spines, the thoracic spine creates a natural backward curvature called a *kyphosis*. This completes a springy 'S' shape, which gives the spine its load-bearing capabilities. It is therefore a perfectly natural curve that varies between individuals; however, as discussed in the case of the cervical spine, the lumbar curve can be exaggerated with poor posture. The effects of increased postural loads will be explained in more detail in the section on common spinal problems.

Lumbar Spine

The lumbar spine forms the lowest part of the mobile spine regions and sits on the sacral bones. Its natural forward curvature, known as the *lumbar lordosis*, is a secondary curve that forms in humans once we begin to walk. Comprising five vertebral bones and intervening intervertebral discs, the chunky lumbar spine reflects its load-bearing role, as can be seen in Figure 11.6.

The facet joints in this spinal region are oriented in such a way as to limit rotation, which was more freely available in the thoracic spine. The lumbar spine, however, has at its disposal a good range of flexion and extension movements, which are ultimately restrained by the discs and ligaments. Sustained extremes of lumbar spine flexion due to postural strain will stress the lumbar discs and ligaments, causing them to *creep*. This is a term commonly used in material sciences to describe the tendency for solid structures to deform under prolonged stress. The results of this phenomenon will be explored further when we discuss common lower back problems.

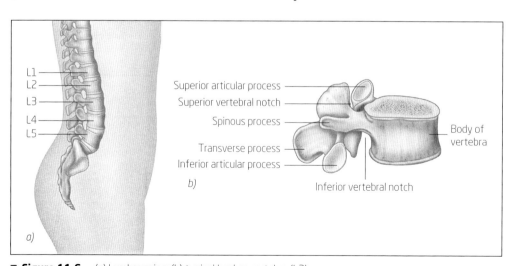

■ **Figure 11.6.** (a) Lumbar spine; (b) typical lumbar vertebra (L3).

KEY POINT *Lumbar spinal discs and ligaments can slowly deform under sustained loads, such as poor posture. Prevention is better than cure, so work on good posture and avoid prolonged postures.*

There are five pairs of spinal nerves in the lumbar spine, which exit at their corresponding levels on either side of the bony spinal column. These nerve roots can supply various sections of the buttocks and legs, down to the feet and toes. The nerves can be susceptible to mechanical irritation as they travel within the bony spinal column or as they exit it. If you have symptoms of pain, changes in sensation, or weakness of the legs, we strongly recommend that you seek qualified health or medical advice before commencing any corrective exercise, including body-weight exercise.

In the absence of these symptoms, some common causes of spinal pain and dysfunction will now be examined, along with some body-weight exercises to condition and rehabilitate the spine.

■ Common Spinal Dysfunction

Postural Dysfunction of the Neck

We have already discussed several functions of the spinal column, from providing support and movement, to protecting the internal organs of the chest. The spinal column also houses the spinal cord, which connects the body with the brain. The neck, however, has one crucial function that we should not overlook – it must position the head in such a way that our senses can operate effectively. Take a moment to think about how you position your head in order to hear a faint sound or to adjust your visual field. And what about the inner ear, which maintains your balance? A poorly positioned head means major disruption to this delicate balance system.

KEY POINT *The neck must position itself in such a way that it sustains the ability of the head to operate the senses of vision and hearing, and also to maintain balance, effectively.*

When the rest of your spine is slumped in a poor posture, the neck must then make up the difference in order for the head to maintain its position. This is often the basis of cervical spine postural dysfunction. It is a relatively common condition, causing pain in the neck when there is no significant trauma or tissue damage.

Adopting poor spinal postures over a prolonged period of time is the main cause of this condition. This can be any position, but more often than not it involves the modern-day curses of sitting, watching television, driving a car or using a computer. Increasingly sedentary lifestyles or working patterns can therefore lead to muscle weakness and lengthening, while other muscles at the neck and shoulders become tight and overactive.

An example of how these muscle imbalances can develop is given in Figure 11.7, which

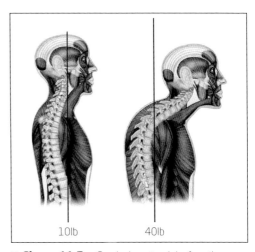

10lb   40lb

■ **Figure 11.7.** Cervical postural dysfunction.

shows a posture that increases the load of the head by more than three times its normal weight. This load can be as much as 20kg, or 45lb! Just imagine this extra stress on your neck structures every day!

KEY EXERCISE 11.1: NECK RETRACTION

Target Area: Cervical spine
Sets: 2
Reps: 10
Rest: 20 seconds   **LEVEL 1**

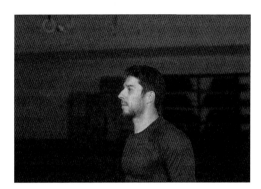

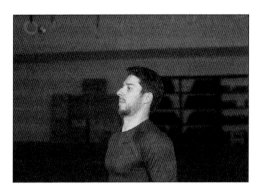

The neck retraction is great for addressing the problem of a pronounced postural lordosis in the neck.

1. To perform the neck retraction, stand up in a relaxed position.

2. Allow the neck and head to settle into a neutral position. Draw your shoulders gently away from your ears and imagine your neck lengthening.

3. Now move your chin directly backwards in a horizontal plane. You should feel your neck muscles below your jaw tense gently in effort. Feel the stretch at the base of your skull and at the back of the neck.

4. Hold this position for a few seconds, and then return your head to the starting position. This counts as one repetition.

Teaching Points

The main issue with the neck retraction exercise is not moving the head directly backwards, but rather tilting or pivoting it in order to lower the chin. To resolve this issue, it can help to film yourself performing the exercise, or get a friend or training partner to watch you.

Postural Dysfunction of the Thoracic Spine

Postural dysfunction, or postural syndrome, can also affect the upper back (thoracic spine) and is a relatively common cause of pain in this region of the spine in the absence of any trauma. If you are experiencing pain from postural syndrome, this will mainly occur while doing activities that place prolonged stress on your otherwise normal spinal structures.

Postural syndrome in the upper back occurs in a similar fashion to the cervical spine, through sitting or standing in poor positions for prolonged periods of time. This may even include sports such as cycling or hockey.

With prolonged sitting or standing, the thoracic spine can begin to slouch under the effects of gravity. The thoracic kyphosis increases, and as the ribcage slumps, the shoulder blades slide forwards, causing the shoulders to round. The neck must now increase its lordosis posture to compensate for the thoracic spine, because otherwise your line of sight would angle towards the floor. Try it for yourself and see what happens when you do not adapt the posture at the neck. Before too long, you will begin to realise why upper back, neck and shoulder pain and dysfunction occur. We have not even started on the lower back yet!

> **KEY POINT** *As the thoracic kyphosis increases with postural stress, the shoulders slump forwards and become rounded and the neck lordosis must increase in order to compensate.*

KEY EXERCISE 11.2: UPPER SPINE FOAM ROLL

Target Area: Thoracic spine
Sets: 3
Duration: 30 seconds
Rest: 30 seconds   **LEVEL 1**

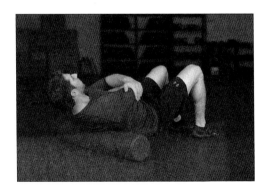

Foam rolling is great for working knotted and sore areas of the targeted muscles. Your body

weight is used to massage the sore areas. By the very nature of the body position, this exercise will reduce the thoracic kyphosis and unload that postural strain!

1. To perform the upper spine foam roll, sit down on the ground with the foam roller behind you.
2. Lie back onto the roller so that it is positioned across the lower parts of your shoulder blades. Raise your hips off the ground. Plant your feet with bent knees.
3. Wrap your arms around you so that your back is rounded. This will make it easier to target the middle spine and ribs.
4. Roll backwards and forwards slowly, starting from the top of your back and moving down to just above the lower back. If there are any sore areas, pay particular attention to these parts. Roll for 30 seconds and then rest. While resting, you may find that you get a beneficial stretch by allowing the middle spine to arch over the foam roller.

Teaching Points

When first starting to foam roll, you will need to use a soft foam roller, as this will be the least painful. As you progress, you can move on to harder rollers, which will support the spine more and apply firmer pressure to the soft tissues.

Rib Joint Dysfunction (Thoracic Spine)

Rib joint dysfunction has been regarded as a potentially common problem that involves poor joint stability where the ribs meet the thoracic spine. The joints here are relatively shallow, making them susceptible to mechanical over-stressing. Pain is often sudden, sometimes after working in a rotated-spine position. Deep breathing, stretching the spine backwards and performing rotational spinal movements may worsen the pain. Such a problem can be a result of underlying poor postural habits, as explained above. Symptoms often settle after a few days. To reduce the chance of recurrence, and to ease the pain associated with this condition, we offer Key Exercise 11.3.

KEY EXERCISE 11.3: UPPER BACK STRETCH

Target Area: Thoracic and cervical spines
Sets: 3
Duration: 20 seconds each side
Rest: 30 seconds   **LEVEL 1**

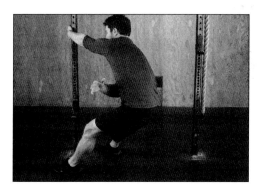

Stretching the muscles of the upper back is important in view of modern-day postures. In addition to stretching the muscles of the back, this exercise will also provide some gentle traction to the middle spine and the ribs. The stretching exercise for the upper back is simple and effective, and can be performed almost anywhere.

1. To perform the upper back stretch, hold onto a solid object. If you are in a gym, a bar or frame of some sort will be perfect,

provided it cannot move. If you are at home, a doorframe or any other solid object will suffice.
2. Keep the working arm straight, and wrap your free arm around yourself.
3. Now lean back, keeping your feet flat on the ground and dropping your hips if necessary. You may need to twist your body slightly in order to transfer the stretch to all areas of the muscle.
4. Hold the stretch for 20 seconds, and then switch sides and repeat.

Teaching Points

If you experience any natural popping or clicking of the spine with this exercise, please be reassured that this is quite normal. Do not force your spine to make these noises, though; if they occur naturally during a stretch, then that is fine.

Try this exercise along with Key Exercise 11.2 for a more effective approach to this problem.

Thoracic Disc Dysfunction

Thoracic disc dysfunction is a less common condition and will therefore be covered only briefly here. Some reports in the literature suggest a rate of one in a thousand, while others have proposed one in a million. When the condition is minor and uncomplicated, intermittent thoracic pain may be experienced, usually in the lower region, and is worse with sitting, rotating or side-bending. There may even be some pain around the chest or from the back to the front. In these situations, we suggest trying Key Exercise 11.4.

If there are signs of changes in control and sensation of the legs, bladder or bowel, we recommend urgent medical attention.

KEY EXERCISE 11.4: COBRA STRETCH

Target Area: Thoracic and lumbar spines
Sets: 3
Duration: 10–20 seconds
Rest: 30 seconds

LEVEL 1

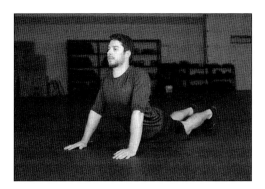

The cobra stretch is designed to target the lower abdominal muscles, and to stretch through the thoracic and lumbar spines. It is a good stretch to perform if you have a low level of spinal flexibility, and also if you have been doing some demanding core exercise.

1. To perform the cobra stretch, lie face down with your hands flat on the floor. Stretch your legs out behind you.
2. Push up with your arms, keeping your hips in contact with the ground. Curl your spine and look up at the ceiling until you feel the stretch in your back or abdominal muscles.
3. Try to extend your elbows to maximise the stretch. If you are able, you can breathe out as you arch backwards in order to increase the stretch a little at a time. Hold this position for 10–20 seconds, and then release slowly and rest.

Teaching Points

If you are not strong enough to support yourself with your arms, you can perform this stretch by supporting yourself on your forearms.

Lower Back Pain

Most lower back pain is non-serious in nature and is likely to improve over time, with the possibility of intermittent pain flare-ups. Some research suggests that up to 35% of the UK adult population will suffer back pain at any one time, with up to 80% of the same population experiencing some back pain over their lifetime. It is therefore reasonable to say that back pain is a common occurrence in the human life span. Some might even suggest that it is 'normal' for it to occur at some point within the human lifetime according to the statistics. That said, there are some causes of back pain that are more serious; if you are in any doubt, you should see a qualified health or medical professional.

The following sections will deal with non-serious and common causes of lower back pain that have the potential to respond very well to physical activity. Accordingly, we will suggest some appropriate body-weight exercises for you to consider.

Nonspecific Lower Back Pain

Nonspecific lower back pain or *simple lower back pain* are common terms for lower back pain that is non-serious and has no clear single cause with regard to the pain and dysfunction being experienced. The majority of cases of this type of back pain improve within four months, although it is acknowledged that pain can persist in some for up to a year. What we hope has become clear so far in this book is that the human musculoskeletal system is incredibly complex, and the spine is probably the best example of this with all of its intricate structures. From reading other parts of this book, you will also have noticed that we have avoided the use of specific diagnostic titles in many areas; you will have seen that we have justified this position from a perspective of increased knowledge of human pain. You may need to read that last sentence again – we know more about pain now than we have ever done in the past, yet we use less specific diagnostic terminology for many musculoskeletal problems. Nonspecific back pain is a prime example of this, and we will now explain why in relation to the pain you may be experiencing.

Any structure in the lumbar spine that is supplied by nerves (which is most of it) can cause symptoms of lower back pain and even referred pain to the buttocks, legs or feet. This long list of potential pain-causing structures has already been highlighted in the spine anatomy and briefly includes the muscles, ligaments, nerve roots, facet joints, discs, vertebral bones and even the connective tissue that wraps around nearly everything else in the spine.

At this point you are probably thinking, 'Yes, but wouldn't a scan of my spine show which of these structures is causing my pain?' Unless there is a single serious cause of your back pain, which is less common, the answer is, 'No, it wouldn't.' For example, evidence of a herniated disc has been observed with medical imaging, such as CT and MRI scans, in 20% to 75% of people with no sciatic pain. This means that some people with disc problems will have back pain, while others with similar-looking disc problems on the medical imaging pictures will have no symptoms.

If you have nonspecific or simple lower back pain and you have been checked by a medical or health professional, you may benefit from 'nonspecific' body-weight exercises that stretch and strengthen your spine and other body areas. Over time, these exercises will condition you to move better

and to withstand the physical stresses and strains of modern living. We recommend Key Exercises 11.4 and 11.5, but if you currently have little or no lower back pain, try the body-weight winner Key Exercise 11.5.

KEY EXERCISE 11.5: PLANK

Target Area: Thoracic and lumbar spines
Sets: 3
Duration: 10–60 seconds, depending on ability
Rest: 30 seconds **LEVEL 1**

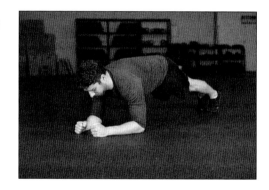

Perhaps the simplest and most effective exercise for the core, and therefore the spine, is the plank. The plank consists of holding the body horizontally, with support on the forearms and toes. The main areas worked by this exercise are the muscles supporting the thoracic and lumbar spine. It is a great introductory exercise that can be expanded in many ways.

1. To perform the plank, place your forearms on the ground. Stretch your legs out behind you and balance on your toes.
2. Make sure that your upper arms are vertical, and then raise your hips up until they are level with your shoulders. Your back should be as straight as possible, with no sagging of the lower back.

3. If you feel a pinching or straining sensation in the lower back, try to tuck your tailbone under in order to reduce the pressure here and to maintain a stronger and more neutral spine position.

Teaching Points

If this version of the plank is too difficult, you can make it easier by resting on your knees instead of your toes; this will reduce the amount of body weight being supported by the core. You can also rest your arms on a raised platform to move more of your body weight onto the lower body.

Lumbar Disc and Joint Degenerative Changes

Generally speaking, this is a problem more likely to be seen in the older age group, and is a gradual change in the mobility of the facet joints of the spine and the movement available due to the intervertebral discs (Figure 11.8). If you start to develop a stiff spine suddenly or at a relatively young age, we suggest that you have an assessment by a suitably qualified health or medical professional.

You may have noticed that your spinal movements have gradually stiffened and eventually given rise to lower back pain with no recent injury. If you find that bending forwards is relatively easy, but straightening your spine or flexing to the sides is more difficult or uncomfortable, then you could be suffering from degenerative changes to the spinal column. This may or may not show on x-rays of the spine; moreover, studies have found degenerative changes on spinal x-rays in the absence of lower back pain. If you have been advised by a qualified health or medical professional to exercise and mobilise your spine, we recommend Key Exercise 11.6.

KEY EXERCISE 11.6: STANDING SIDE STRETCH

Target Area: Thoracic and lumbar spines
Sets: 3 each side
Duration: 20 seconds each side
Rest: 30 seconds   **LEVEL 1**

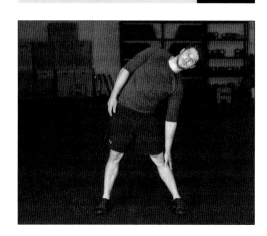

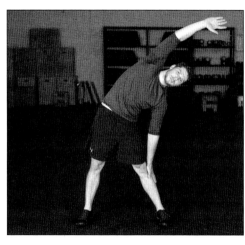

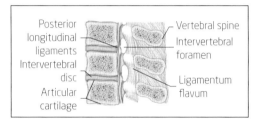

■ **Figure 11.8.** Anatomy of the lumbar spine and the intervertebral disc.

The standing side stretch is designed to increase the mobility in both the thoracic and the lumbar spine. You will feel a stretch in the oblique muscles and possibly around the spine itself. The oblique muscles at the sides of the core aid in bending and twisting motions, and may have tightened because of a stiff spine.

1. To perform the standing side stretch, stand with your feet shoulder-width apart and your arms by your sides.
2. Bend at the waist and start to slide one hand down your side. You should feel the stretch in the extended side of your core.
3. Keep going until you reach the limit of your mobility. Hold the stretch for 20 seconds, change sides and repeat.

Teaching Points

If you find that this method does not give you a sufficiently satisfying stretch, you can raise one arm and reach over to the side of your torso. Reaching with the arm in this way will also help maintain or develop shoulder mobility.

■ Body-weight Exercises for Improved Spine Function

The following exercises have been put together to assist you in further alleviating back and neck pain, or to help develop a resilient and injury-resistant spine.

EXERCISE 11.7: LOWER SPINE FOAM ROLL

Target Area: Lumbar spine
Sets: 3
Duration: 10–30 seconds, depending on tolerance
Rest: 30 seconds   **LEVEL 1**

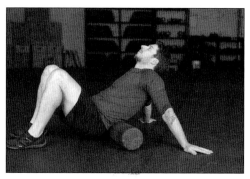

Continuing our look at spinal foam rolling, we arrive at the lumbar spine. Many factors can contribute to lower back pain, some of which may be muscular in origin. Foam rolling is a great way to 'iron out' some of that muscular tension.

1. To perform the lower spine foam roll, sit down on the ground with the foam roller behind you.
2. Lie back onto the roller so that it is positioned across your lower back. In order to create the pressure against the low back, you may need to slightly raise your hips off the ground. Plant your feet with bent knees.
3. Place your arms on the ground behind you, supporting your weight.
4. Roll backwards and forwards slowly, concentrating on the bottom of your back. After you have rolled for around 20 seconds, pause at the bottom of your spine and allow your back to curl over the foam roller. Hold this position for 10–30 seconds.

Teaching Points

As before, if you are just starting to foam roll, you will want to begin with a soft foam roller. This will be less uncomfortable and will allow you to build up to harder rollers.

EXERCISE 11.8: CAT STRETCH

Target Area: Thoracic, cervical and lumbar spines
Sets: 3
Duration: 30 seconds
Rest: 30 seconds

LEVEL 1

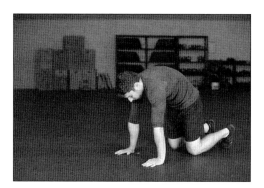

For anybody who has mobility or flexibility issues with the thoracic area of the spine, the cat stretch is a good starting point. It is a stretch that is often seen in yoga and other flexibility programs, and is an essential exercise in our bulletproof program.

1. To perform the cat stretch, get down onto your hands and knees. Your arms and thighs should be vertical. Your neck should be relaxed and your eyes looking down.
2. From here, push your spine up towards the ceiling. Think about separating your shoulder blades and tucking your tailbone under.
3. Push up as far as you can, and then hold for 30 seconds.

Teaching Points

Moving the spine in this way can be difficult, especially if you are struggling to know what muscles to use to make the movement happen. To help with this, try arching your back and sticking your buttocks out first, and then push your spine up towards the ceiling. You will find that this helps to activate the opposing muscle groups, and you will be able to feel which muscles to use. You will also develop better awareness of your spinal posture.

EXERCISE 11.9: SKYDIVER

Target Area: Thoracic and lumbar spines
Sets: 3
Duration: 20 seconds
Rest: 30 seconds

LEVEL 2

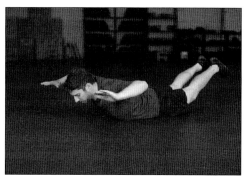

The skydiver exercise works the extensor muscles of the lower back and develops active extension of the lumbar spine. Many people might struggle with this movement, because the muscles running down the spine (the erector spinae group) are weak in many of us. It is very important to strengthen these muscles to support proper spinal function.

1. To perform the skydiver, lie face down with your arms out in front of you, elbows bent at 90 degrees.
2. Now use the muscles of your back to raise your legs and your upper body off the ground. The muscles of the upper

and middle back will work to hold the upper body off the floor, while the lumbar muscles of the lower back will work to hold the legs off the floor.

3. Raise your upper and lower body off the ground as far as you can, and then hold this position for 20 seconds.

Teaching Points

When performing the skydiver, think about squeezing all of the muscles of the back, including the buttocks; this will ensure that you get the maximum benefit out of the movement. In addition, try not to bounce, and stay as still as possible once in the skydiver position. Try also not to strain the hamstrings at the backs of your thighs.

EXERCISE 11.10: SIDE PLANK

Target Area: Thoracic and lumbar spines
Sets: 2
Duration: 10–60 seconds each side
Rest: 30 seconds

LEVEL 2

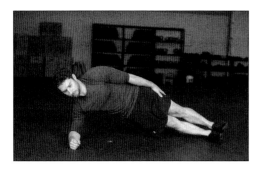

Although the plank works the core very well, the demand on the muscles in the sides of the core (the obliques) is much less. To target these muscles more effectively, we can perform the side plank; this uses the same principle as the plank, in that the body is held

rigid, using gravity as the resistance. The key here is to hold a good 'neutral' spinal posture against the force of gravity.

1. To perform the side plank, lie on your side with your lower forearm flat on the floor, at 90 degrees to your body.
2. Place both legs together with one foot on top of the other.
3. From here, raise your hips into the air, until a straight line can be drawn through your shoulders, hips, knees and ankles. Place your free arm by your side, in the air, or touching the ground to help with balance.
4. Keeping your head and neck neutral, hold this position for the required time, and then rest and repeat on the opposite side.

Teaching Points

The side plank should be manageable for short lengths of time, even for those who have not trained before. If you do find it difficult to perform, you can adapt it in the same way as the normal plank, by resting on the knees instead of the feet; this reduces the proportion of weight supported by the core, and therefore makes the exercise easier.

EXERCISE 11.11: SIDE LEAN

Target Area: Thoracic and lumbar spines
Sets: 3
Reps: 10 (5 each side)
Rest: 20 seconds

LEVEL 1

The side lean helps to strengthen the lumbar and thoracic spines, and aids in working on any poor side-leaning postures you may have developed. The exercise will help to increase the flexibility of your spine as well. For this

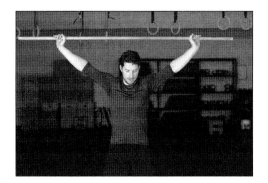

2. From here, bend over to one side at the waist, controlling the movement using the muscles in the sides of your core. Keep your arms straight at all times, and do not allow your shoulders to move towards your head; the movement must come just from your waist.

3. Once you have leant as far as you can, return to the upright position and repeat on the other side. This counts as one repetition.

Teaching Points

The main area that requires attention in this exercise is ensuring that the arms stay straight and relatively static in relation to the head. It is tempting to allow the arms to move independently of the spine, but this is not correct form. Maintaining proper form will make the movement much more effective.

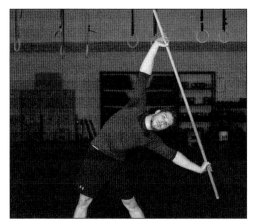

EXERCISE 11.12: REAR SUPPORT

Target Area: Thoracic and lumbar spines, shoulders
Sets: 3
Duration: 10–30 seconds
Rest: 30 seconds   **LEVEL 2**

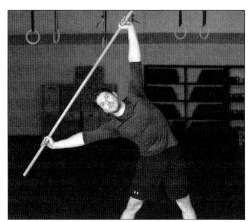

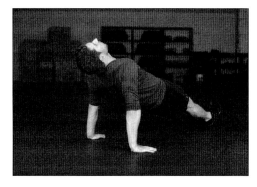

exercise, you will need a light bar, such as a broom handle or exercise barbell.

1. To perform the side lean, grasp the bar with a wide grip and hold it above your head. Stand with your feet wide apart so that your entire body forms a large 'X' shape.

The rear support is another static move that targets most of the muscles of the back, in addition to the shoulders and other muscles of the upper body. All in all, it is a great example of using body-weight exercise to become injury-proof. As an exercise, it is the polar opposite of the plank, and works the opposing muscles groups. It is harder than the plank, mainly because the position is not one that the human body is placed in very often.

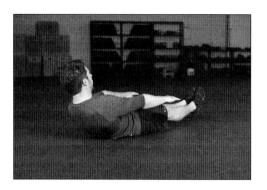

1. To perform the rear support, sit on the ground with your hands flat on the floor, fingers pointing backwards, and your legs straight out in front of you.
2. From here push your hips into the air, keeping your arms straight.
3. Keep pushing your hips up into the air until a straight line can be drawn through your shoulders, hips, knees and ankles. Balance on your heels.
4. Keep your head neutral and neck straight. Hold this position for the required time, and then rest.

Teaching Points

You may find that at first you do not have either the strength to perform the movement, or the shoulder flexibility to allow the position. The bar shoulder dislocate (Chapter 5, Exercise 5.11) will help here, as will the other shoulder stretching exercises. In addition, the exercise can also be performed with the hands resting on a raised platform so that they are higher than the feet. This will make the movement easier to perform, allowing the hands to be moved closer to the ground over time.

EXERCISE 11.13: DISH

Target Area: Thoracic spine, core muscles
Sets: 3
Duration: 20–30 seconds
Rest: 30 seconds   **LEVEL 1**

If the strength of the core is increased, the resilience of the spine to injury is also increased. Developing muscle around the torso, and making the muscles that reside there as resilient as possible, constitute a good course of action for injury prevention. The dish exercise will take your strength to the next level.

1. To perform the dish, lie on your back with your legs straight and your arms by your sides.
2. From here curl your shoulders off the ground and lift your feet and arms about 5cm (2″) into the air at the same time.
3. Keep your pelvis pressed into the ground, while allowing your upper back to rise. To help with this movement, think of trying to curl your body around a large ball.
4. Hold this position for the required time, and then rest.

Teaching Points

Although it looks like it might be easy, the dish is a tough exercise and much trickier to perform properly than the plank. To make it easier, you can bend your knees to bring the weight of your legs closer to your centre of gravity; if you do this, make sure that your feet stay close to the ground, with only your knees bending. As you progress, extend your legs until they are straight.

EXERCISE 11.14: BRIDGE

Target Area: Spine, buttocks, hips
Sets: 3
Duration: 10–20 seconds
Rest: 30 seconds

LEVEL 3

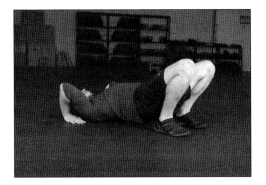

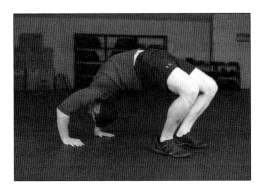

One of the best movements for spinal health is the bridge, or 'back bend'; this type of movement is used in gymnastics, calisthenics and even yoga. Another bulletproof classic, the bridge is more difficult to perform than many movements in this book, but the benefits cannot be overstated. As this exercise is so tough, not just strengthwise but also in terms of mobility and flexibility, take your time with it.

1. To perform the bridge, lie down on your back and bend your knees so that your feet are flat on the floor. Make sure that your feet are not too far away from your buttocks, but not too close either.
2. Lift your arms into the air and place your palms on the ground, fingers pointing towards your feet. This position will require good shoulder and wrist flexibility; if this is lacking, you should spend time on the relevant exercises in Chapters 5 and 7 of this book.
3. Making sure that your hands and feet are firmly planted, try to push your torso into the air. Use all of the muscles of your back to do this, while straightening your arms and legs as much as possible.
4. Once you have pushed your torso up as high as possible, hold the position for the required amount of time, and then rest.

Teaching Points

There is no doubt that the bridge is one of the most difficult exercises in this chapter; for this reason, make sure that you only attempt it when you are ready. In terms of making the movement easier, this can be achieved by moving the hands and feet further apart. As your flexibility and strength increase, you can move your hands and feet closer together, which will place more demand on the flexibility and mobility of the spine and shoulders.

EXERCISE 11.15: EXTENDED PLANK

Target Area: Thoracic and lumbar spines, core muscles
Sets: 3
Duration: 5–15 seconds
Rest: 30 seconds

LEVEL 3

If you have mastered the plank and want to take your strength to the next level, you can

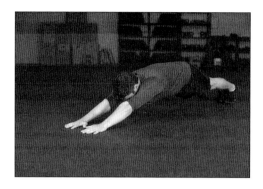

try the extended plank. This is a variable exercise, in that it can be made more or less difficult depending on your strength. In terms of equipment, make sure that the floor you perform this movement on is as non-slip as possible.

1. To perform the extended plank, assume a standard push-up position. Your hands should be shoulder-width apart and your arms vertical, and you should be balancing on your toes.
2. Now walk your hands forwards slowly until you feel the muscles in your core working to hold the position.
3. Keep your neck and head neutral and arms straight, and hold the position for as long as you can, aiming for 15 seconds.

Teaching Points

The extended plank is an exercise with great scope. If you need to make this exercise easier, move your hands and feet closer together; if you need to make it more difficult, move them further apart. The end goal of this movement is to hold the position with the chest and torso very close to, but not touching, the ground; this will stress the spine and the core, building high levels of strength and injury resistance.

■ Goal Exercises for the Spine

As in the case of other body parts, the spine and core have their own goal exercises; these are designed to test and build overall strength and mobility, and will give you a clear picture of how your core strength and spinal mobility are progressing. The movements can also be used as exercises in their own right, as part of a larger routine, or once you need a greater challenge in your workouts.

GOAL EXERCISE 11.16: KNEELING ROLL-OUT

Target Area: Thoracic and lumbar spines
Sets: 3
Reps: 5–10
Rest: 45 seconds   **LEVEL 3**

The kneeling roll-out is an extremely tough but useful exercise, but is nowhere near as popular or well known as it ought to be. The reason for both the difficulty and the benefits of this exercise is that the core is forced to keep the spine in a stable position while exerting tremendous amounts of force. This means that the kneeling roll-out differs from movements such as sit-ups and crunches, which *shorten* the length of the torso. This exercise, which requires an abdominal wheel, will develop strength and injury resistance while working with the spine as a long lever.

1. To perform the kneeling roll-out, get down onto your knees and hold the abdominal wheel with both hands.
2. Ensure that your elbows are straight, your spine is horizontal and your thighs are vertical. This is the starting and finishing position.

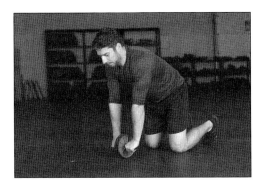

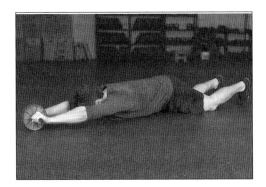

3. Begin to roll the wheel forwards, keeping your arms and legs at the same relative angle throughout the movement.
4. Keep the head and neck position neutral, and roll forwards until your chest touches the ground. Pause for a second, and then reverse the movement until you arrive back in the starting position. This counts as one repetition.

Teaching Points

As the kneeling roll-out is such a tough exercise, most people will have to make the movement easier in order to progress with it. Rolling the abdominal wheel into a wall or other solid object can help here. To use this method, assume the starting position, with the abdominal wheel a small distance away from the base of the wall or a solid, stationary object. Roll forwards until the wheel stops against the wall, and then use your core muscles to roll back again. Begin with the wheel close to the wall and move steadily further away until you can perform the kneeling roll-out with no assistance.

GOAL EXERCISE 11.17: HANGING LEG RAISE

Target Area: Thoracic spine
Sets: 3
Reps: 5–10
Rest: 45 seconds

LEVEL 3

The hanging leg raise is an excellent test of core strength, while also encouraging spinal mobility in the same exercise. It is a standard movement in gymnastic circles, and uses the weight of the lower body as the resistance. You will need a pull-up bar or gymnastic rings.

1. Grab onto a pull-up bar with an overhand grip; the hands should be shoulder-width apart or slightly wider.
2. Hang with a straight body and straight legs, with the scapulae engaged and the shoulders pulled down.
3. Contract your core muscles and begin to raise your legs into the air, bending at the waist. Pull down hard with your upper body to stop any momentum.

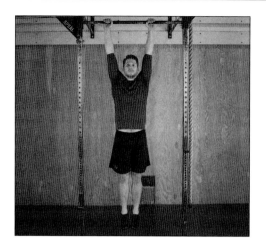

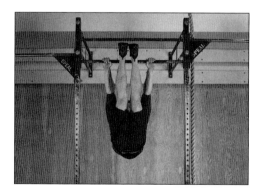

Teaching Points

If the full version of the hanging leg raise is too difficult for you, it can be made easier by doing a hanging knee raise; this is performed in exactly the same way, except that the knees are bent and brought up to the chest, instead of the legs being kept straight. With your knees bent, more of your body weight is kept closer to your centre of gravity, and so the resistance that the core muscles are working against will feel much less. As your core strength increases, you can progress to straightening your legs a little at a time.

Another issue that can affect one's ability to perform the leg raise is a lack of flexibility in the hamstrings. To remedy this, spend time on increasing flexibility in this area, most notably with the hamstring stretch (Key Exercise 8.3).

GOAL EXERCISE 11.18: ARCH-UP

Target Area: Thoracic and lumbar spines
Sets: 3
Reps: 10
Rest: 30 seconds

LEVEL 2

One goal exercise that concentrates on the lumbar spine is the arch-up. This is an extension of the skydiver exercise, and requires the arms and legs to be stretched out from your centre of gravity.

4. Keep raising your legs until they are at least horizontal. You may even strive to reach a higher position, to touch your hands with your toes!

5. Pause for a second, and then return your legs to the starting position, always under control.

1. To perform the arch-up, lie face down with your arms stretched out in front of you and your legs straight behind you. This is the starting position.

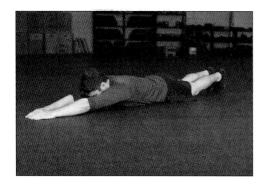

2. From here, raise your arms and legs into the air at the same time, contracting the muscles in your back.
3. Keep raising your arms and legs as far as possible, aiming to get them well into the air.
4. Pause for a second, and then return your arms and legs to the starting position. This counts as one repetition.

Teaching Points

For many people, the arch-up should not pose too much of a problem; the real challenge is in developing enough strength and mobility to raise the upper body and legs high into the air. This is something that will develop with time. Stick with it!

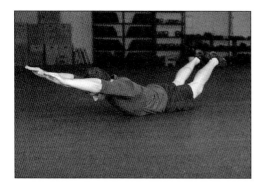

12

Upper Body Training Programs

Note: *It is worth reiterating that the training programs outlined over the next few chapters are guides only, and not every part of every program will be applicable to every reader. For example, if you have a particular shoulder injury, you may be able to perform the shoulder exercises only at the beginner level, but the lower body and spinal exercises at the advanced level. This is normal and should be expected in these situations.*

Now that you have an idea of the anatomy of each joint, and are familiar with the injuries that can occur and the exercises that will help to build injury prevention in each area, it is time to look at various training programs. These guides will consolidate all of this knowledge in a structured way that you can follow in your training sessions and workouts.

▨ Upper Body: Beginner Program

The upper body program actually consists of three separate programs, divided into beginner, intermediate and advanced levels

of ability. The beginner program can be seen in Table 12.1. Notice that the name of the exercise, the number of sets, the number of repetitions or the duration, and the amount of rest time is included for ease of use.

■ **Table 12.1.** Upper body: beginner program.

	Sets	Reps/ duration	Rest
Wrist exercises			
Forearm and wrist stretch 1	3	20 seconds	20 seconds
Forearm and wrist stretch 2	3	20 seconds	20 seconds
Push-up support	3	20 seconds	20 seconds
Elbow exercises			
Inverted-wrist wall push-up	3	5–20, depending on strength	30 seconds
Ledge dip	3	10	45 seconds
Arm rotation	3	10	20 seconds
Shoulder exercises			
Chest stretch	3	15 seconds	10 seconds
Shoulder stretch	3	15 seconds	10 seconds
Rotator cuff stretch	3	10 seconds	10 seconds
Scapula foam roll	3	10 seconds	30–45 seconds

As you can see, in this beginner program there are exercises for the wrist, elbow and shoulder. Ideally you will follow the program from top to bottom, performing each exercise for the required number of sets and repetitions before moving on to the next exercise, progressing all the way down the table until you finish. A program like this will be extremely beneficial if you introduce it into your routine. As it will not take a huge amount of time, it is possible to perform this program three to five times a week without it impacting on your life too much.

In your weekly training schedule, you will need some rest days, and so a week in which you train three times might be as follows:

Monday:	Train
Tuesday:	Rest
Wednesday:	Train
Thursday:	Rest
Friday:	Train
Saturday:	Rest
Sunday:	Rest

This method can be followed for the other programs set out in Chapters 12, 13, 14 and 15.

▦ Upper Body: Intermediate Program

Once you have some experience with the beginner program, or when the exercises in it do not present much of a challenge, you can move on to the intermediate program (Table 12.2), which is suitable for those with intermediate ability. These exercises will still work the same joints and muscles, though in slightly different ways, but the benefits

■ **Table 12.2.** Upper body: intermediate program.

	Sets	Reps/ duration	Rest
Wrist exercises			
Fist push-up support	3	20 seconds	30 seconds
Fingertip push-up support	3	10–20 seconds	30 seconds
Elbow exercises			
Forklift	3	5–10, depending on strength	30 seconds
Planche lean	3	10 seconds	30 seconds
Shoulder exercises			
Dead hang	3	20 seconds	30 seconds
Scapula push-up	3	10	30 seconds
Band shoulder dislocate	3	10	20 seconds

will nevertheless be felt. Again, as there are a limited number of exercises specified, this entire program can be performed three to five times a week comfortably, with rest days inserted in between your training days.

▦ Upper Body: Advanced Program

Once the exercises in the intermediate program become too easy, or if you are looking for more variation and a greater challenge, you can move on to the advanced program (Table 12.3), which contains exercises suitable for advanced exercisers. The same method should be followed here: perform all of the exercises (if possible), for the required number of sets, number of repetitions or duration, and rest times, until you have worked your way through the table and completed all of the exercises. Again, as there are only eight exercises here, performing the program three to five times a week is possible, and recommended.

■ **Table 12.3.** Upper body: advanced program.

	Sets	Reps/ duration	Rest
Wrist exercises			
Inverted-wrist push-up support	3	10–20 seconds	45 seconds
False-grip hang	3	10–20 seconds	45 seconds
Kneeling inverted-wrist push-up	3	5	45 seconds
Elbow exercises			
Pull-up/static hang	3	1–20, depending on strength	45 seconds
Negative chin-up	3	3–10	45 seconds
Shoulder exercises			
Scapula dip	3	10	30 seconds
Frog stance	3	10 seconds	30 seconds
Scapula pull-up	3	10	30 seconds

13

Lower Body Training Programs

The lower body is home to many potential injuries, from sprains and strains of the ankle, to ligament issues in the knee and dysfunctions of the hip. The programs we have devised here will help in all aspects of injury prevention and rehabilitation of the lower body, regardless of your level of ability or your current injury status.

■ Lower Body: Beginner Program

The beginner program for the lower body (Table 13.1) is designed to get you moving again after a long time away from physical training, or when you are too injured to perform many of the strength-building movements. Accordingly, the exercises in this program revolve around mobility and flexibility, with the chief aim being to restore movement in preparation for more demanding exercises.

As with the programs for the other parts of the body, this program should ideally be followed and performed from start to finish, beginning at the top of the table and working your way down until all of the exercises are

■ **Table 13.1.** Lower body: beginner program.

	Sets	Reps/ duration	Rest
Hip exercises			
Knee circle	3	10 each leg	10 seconds
Hamstring stretch	3	20 seconds each leg	20 seconds
Hip flexor stretch	3	20 seconds each leg	20 seconds
Knee exercises			
ITB mobilisation	3	20–30 seconds	20 seconds
Adductor foam roll	3	30 seconds each leg	20 seconds
Quadriceps stretch	3	30 seconds each leg	20 seconds
Gym ball hamstring curl	3	10	20 seconds
Ankle exercises			
Unloaded dorsiflexion	3	10 each leg	20 seconds
Unloaded plantar flexion	3	10 each leg	20 seconds
Unloaded inversion	3	10 each leg	20 seconds
Unloaded eversion	3	10 each leg	20 seconds
Calf stretch	3	20 seconds	20 seconds

completed. If for any reason you cannot perform any of the exercises, leave them out and only do the ones you can. As your injury gets better, or your strength or mobility increases, you can then introduce the other exercises.

As regards training frequency, again this program can be performed three to five times a week with very little disruption to your daily life. In your weekly training schedule, you will need some rest days, and so a week in which you train three times might be as follows:

Monday:	Train
Tuesday:	Rest
Wednesday:	Train
Thursday:	Rest
Friday:	Train
Saturday:	Rest
Sunday:	Rest

■ Lower Body: Intermediate Program

Once the beginner program becomes too easy, or you need to inject some strength movements into your routine, this intermediate program will be where to start (Table 13.2). Some of the movements in this program are stretching and mobility based (e.g. the groin stretch and ITB foam roll) and some are strength based (e.g. the squat and the lunge).

As before, the idea is to run through the table of exercises, performing each for the required number of sets and repetitions (or specified duration) until they are finished. If you unable to perform any of the exercises for any reason, leave them out until you are capable of doing so. Regarding frequency, three to five times a week will give great returns.

■ **Table 13.2.** Lower body: intermediate program.

	Sets	Reps/ duration	Rest
Hip exercises			
Deep squat position	3	30 seconds	20 seconds
Groin stretch	3	20 seconds	20 seconds
Glute stretch	3	20 seconds each leg	20 seconds
Knee exercises			
V-up with ball squeeze	3	5–10	30 seconds
Squat	3	15–20	45 seconds
ITB foam roll	3	30 seconds each leg	30 seconds
Lunge	3	10 each leg	30 seconds
Ankle exercises			
Anterior tibial muscle stretch	3	30 seconds	20 seconds
Downward dog	3	30 seconds	30 seconds
Single-leg balance	3	20–60 seconds	30 seconds

■ Lower Body: Advanced Program

When the intermediate program becomes too easy, or the exercises are not serving to increase strength and protect against injury, it will be time to move on to the advanced program (Table 13.3). This contains exercises that will really test your strength (e.g the single-leg squat) and your mobility (e.g. the frog hop). Accordingly, we advise only moving on to this program when you are ready. If you feel like attempting some of the movements beforehand, then go ahead: this is a great way to gauge your progress and see if you are ready for the next step.

As before, the number of exercises here is not excessive and will allow you to perform the program three to five times a week, and to also add in other programs from the upper body and the spine.

■ **Table 13.3.** Lower body: advanced program.

	Sets	Reps/ duration	Rest
Hip exercises			
Piriformis foam roll and stretch	3	20-30 seconds each leg	30 seconds
Mountain climber	3	10 each leg	30 seconds
Frog hop	3	10	30 seconds
Knee exercises			
Single-leg squat	3	2-5 each leg	30 seconds
Rollover into straddle sit	3	10	30 seconds
Negative hamstring curl	3	2-5	30 seconds
Ankle exercises			
Negative calf raise	3	10-20	30 seconds
Modified frog stance	3	10-20 seconds	30 seconds
Heel sit	3	10-20 seconds	30 seconds

14

Spine Training Programs

The spine and core are very important areas to train, as Chapter 11 hopefully convinced you. Many injuries can occur in the spine and its associated muscles, and so making this area as strong and resilient as possible is a no-brainer. The spine is considered holistically here, and so exercises for each spinal region are presented.

As with the upper body, we have split the exercises for the spine into three distinct programs, namely beginner, intermediate and advanced. These programs will be examined next.

■ Spine: Beginner Program

The beginner program for the spine (Table 14.1) consists of five exercises, which have been chosen to increase mobility and flexibility in the spine, and to get the muscles in the core working. This program is ideal for those who have not trained in a long time (or never), and for those who are coming back from injury and cannot exert much force with their core muscles.

■ **Table 14.1.** Spine: beginner program.

	Sets	Reps/ duration	Rest
Spine exercises			
Upper spine foam roll	3	30 seconds	30 seconds
Upper back stretch	3	20 seconds each side	30 seconds
Cobra stretch	3	20 seconds	30 seconds
Standing side stretch	3	20 seconds each side	30 seconds
Lower spine foam roll	3	30 seconds	30 seconds
Cat stretch	3	30 seconds	30 seconds

As there are only five exercises, it is recommended to perform the entire program as written here, three to five times a week. In addition, it can be combined with the upper body and lower body programs (using the program that is suitable for your ability) in order to create a more rounded routine.

■ Spine: Intermediate Program

Once the beginner program becomes too easy, or if you are looking for more variation, you can move on to the intermediate program

■ **Table 14.2.** Spine: intermediate program.

	Sets	Reps/duration	Rest
Spine exercises			
Skydiver	3	20 seconds	30 seconds
Plank	3	20 seconds	30 seconds
Side lean	3	10 (5 each side)	20 seconds
Side plank	3	20 seconds each side	30 seconds
Neck retraction	2	10	20 seconds

■ **Table 14.3.** Spine: advanced program.

	Sets	Reps/duration	Rest
Spine exercises			
Rear support	3	20 seconds or more	30 seconds
Dish	3	20-30 seconds	30 seconds
Bridge	3	10-20 seconds	30 seconds
Extended plank	3	5-15 seconds	30 seconds

(Table 14.2). This contains some strength-building movements, unlike the beginner program, which is more about stretching and increasing mobility in the spine and core.

■ Spine: Advanced Program

The advanced program (Table 14.3) is what you should move on to after the intermediate program becomes too easy. The exercises in this program can in fact be used as a workout in their own right. The dish, for example, is used in gymnastic programs all over the world, and the extended plank can be made very difficult and used to develop great strength.

15

Full Body Training Programs

Although the body-part-specific training programs are great for those looking to concentrate on a particular body part or injury, it is likely that many people will perform movements for the whole body; indeed, this is something that we highly recommend. If you have an injury just in your shoulder or upper body, it is very good practice to train the spine and the lower body as well; this will both protect against injury in those parts of the body, and avoid any potential imbalances that may result from training only one body part.

■ Full Body: Beginner Program

The full body program for beginners (Table 15.1) is ideal for those who need a rounded routine to start their injury prevention or rehabilitation journey. The exercises here are the same as those in the beginner programs for the specific parts of the body, but now linked together. The idea is that you perform all of the movements for the required sets and repetitions, thus completing the workout. This entire program

■ **Table 15.1.** Full body: beginner program.

	Sets	Reps/ duration	Rest
Wrist exercises			
Forearm stretch 1	3	20 seconds	20 seconds
Forearm stretch 2	3	20 seconds	20 seconds
Push-up support	3	20 seconds	20 seconds
Elbow exercises			
Inverted-wrist wall push-up	3	5–20, depending on strength	30 seconds
Ledge dip	3	10	45 seconds
Arm rotation	3	10	20 seconds
Shoulder exercises			
Chest stretch	3	15 seconds	10 seconds
Shoulder stretch	3	15 seconds	10 seconds
Rotator cuff stretch	3	10 seconds	10 seconds
Scapula foam roll	3	10 seconds	30–45 seconds
Spine exercises			
Upper back stretch	3	20 seconds each side	30 seconds
Upper spine foam roll	3	30 seconds	30 seconds
Cobra stretch	3	20 seconds	30 seconds
Standing side stretch	3	20 seconds	30 seconds
Lower spine foam roll	3	30 seconds	30 seconds
Cat stretch	3	30 seconds	30 seconds

■ **Table 15.1.** Full body: beginner program.

	Sets	Reps/duration	Rest
Hip exercises			
Knee circle	3	10 each leg	10 seconds
Hamstring stretch	3	20 seconds each leg	20 seconds
Hip flexor stretch	3	20 seconds each leg	20 seconds
Knee exercises			
ITB mobilisation	3	20–30 seconds	20 seconds
Adductor foam roll	3	30 seconds each leg	20 seconds
Quadriceps stretch	3	30 seconds each leg	20 seconds
Gym ball hamstring curl	3	10	20 seconds
Ankle exercises			
Unloaded dorsiflexion	3	10 each leg	20 seconds
Unloaded plantar flexion	3	10 each leg	20 seconds
Unloaded inversion	3	10 each leg	20 seconds
Unloaded eversion	3	10 each leg	20 seconds
Calf stretch	3	20 seconds	20 seconds

■ **Table 15.2.** Full body: intermediate program.

	Sets	Reps/duration	Rest
Wrist exercises			
Fist push-up support	3	20 seconds	30 seconds
Fingertip push-up support	3	10–20 seconds	30 seconds
Elbow exercises			
Forklift	3	5–10, depending on strength	30 seconds
Planche lean	3	10 seconds	30 seconds
Shoulder exercises			
Dead hang	3	20 seconds	30 seconds
Scapula push-up	3	10	30 seconds
Band shoulder dislocate	3	10	20 seconds
Spine exercises			
Skydiver	3	20 seconds	30 seconds
Plank	3	20 seconds	30 seconds
Side lean	3	10 (5 each side)	20 seconds
Side plank	3	20 seconds each side	30 seconds
Neck retraction	2	10	20 seconds
Hip exercises			
Deep squat position	3	30 seconds	20 seconds
Groin stretch	3	20 seconds	20 seconds
Glute stretch	3	20 seconds each leg	20 seconds
Knee exercises			
V-up with ball squeeze	3	5–10	30 seconds
Squat	3	15–20	45 seconds
ITB foam roll	3	30 seconds each leg	30 seconds
Lunge	3	10 each leg	30 seconds
Ankle exercises			
Anterior tibial muscle stretch	3	30 seconds	20 seconds
Downward dog	3	30 seconds	30 seconds
Single-leg balance	3	20–60 seconds	30 seconds

should not take more than an hour, and can be performed three to five times a week.

■ Full Body: Intermediate Program

The intermediate program for the full body (Table 15.2) contains more advanced exercises than the beginner program, and it is here that we see more strength-based exercises rather than just stretching and mobility ones. Accordingly, it is important that you take your time with the newer exercises. If some prove too difficult, feel free to insert exercises from the beginner program; this is completely normal and expected, especially if you are recovering from injury or returning after a period of deconditioning.

■ Full Body: Advanced Program

The advanced program for the full body (Table 15.3) contains the most demanding exercises with regard to injury prevention and rehabilitation. As with the other programs in this chapter, the advanced program should be performed three to five times a week in order to get a training effect, with dedicated rest days in between. If you cannot perform some of the movements, feel free to substitute some of the exercises from the intermediate or beginner programs where necessary.

■ **Table 15.3.** Full body: advanced program.

	Sets	Reps/duration	Rest
Wrist exercises			
Inverted-wrist push-up support	3	10–20 seconds	45 seconds
False-grip hang	3	10–20 seconds	45 seconds
Kneeling inverted-wrist push-up	3	5	45 seconds
Elbow exercises			
Pull-up/static hang	3	1–20, depending on strength	45 seconds
Negative chin-up	3	3–10	45 seconds
Shoulder exercises			
Scapula dip	3	10	30 seconds
Frog stance	3	10 seconds	30 seconds
Scapula pull-up	3	10	30 seconds
Spine exercises			
Rear support	3	20 seconds or more	30 seconds
Dish	3	20–30 seconds	30 seconds

	Sets	Reps/duration	Rest
Bridge	3	10–20 seconds	30 seconds
Extended plank	3	5–15 seconds	30 seconds
Hip exercises			
Piriformis foam roll and stretch	3	20–30 seconds each leg	30 seconds
Mountain climber	3	10 each leg	30 seconds
Frog hop	3	10	30 seconds
Knee exercises			
Single-leg squat	3	2–5 each leg	30 seconds
Rollover into straddle sit	3	10	30 seconds
Negative hamstring curl	3	2–5	30 seconds
Ankle exercises			
Negative calf raise	3	10–20	30 seconds
Modified frog stance	3	10–20 seconds	30 seconds
Heel sit	3	10–20 seconds	30 seconds

16
Goal Training Program

By now it should be clear that there are broadly two categories of exercise in this book. The first category consists of the injury prevention and rehabilitation exercises, which cover the major joints of the body, while the second comprises the goal exercises, which are found at the end of each chapter.

As we have said before, the goal exercises are there to help you gauge how you are progressing, and also to act as developmental exercises in their own right. They can also be grouped together to create a more advanced training program. This type of program will contribute further to both preventing and rehabilitating injury, and to increasing your strength, mobility, flexibility and overall physical capacity. In other words, it can be used as a normal workout routine that you can perform for many months, or even years, and also as a precursor to more demanding body-weight exercises.*

*Kalym, A. 2019, *Complete Calisthenics –
The Ultimate Guide to Bodyweight Exercise*, Second Edition, Chichester, UK: Lotus Publishing.

The exercises, sets, repetitions/duration and rest times of the goal program are listed in Table 16.1 for convenience.

■ **Table 16.1.** Goal program.

	Sets	Reps/ duration	Rest
Wrist exercises			
Inverted-wrist push-up	3	10	30 seconds
False-grip pull-up	3	3–5	45 seconds
Fist-supported tuck planche	3	5–20 seconds	45 seconds
Elbow exercises			
Triceps dip	3	5–10	45 seconds
Archer push-up	3	5–10 each side	45 seconds
Shoulder exercises			
Pull-up	3	5–10	45 seconds
German hang	3	15 seconds	30 seconds
Spine exercises			
Kneeling roll-out	3	5–10	45 seconds
Hanging leg raise	3	5–10	45 seconds
Arch-up	3	10	30 seconds
Hip exercises			
Body-weight squat	3	20	45 seconds
Duck walk	3	10–20 steps	45 seconds

(Continued)

■ **Table 16.1.** *(Continued)*

	Sets	Reps/ duration	Rest
Knee exercises			
Ice skater	3	10 (5 each leg)	30 seconds
Jump squat	3	10-15	45 seconds
Jump lunge	3	10-15	45 seconds
Ankle exercises			
Skipping	3	30-60 seconds	45 seconds

All of the movements listed in the goal program will give your body a complete workout, using most muscle groups. As these are body-weight exercises, they will work many muscles simultaneously, to either move the body or support it.

Ideally you should perform all of the exercises here three to five times a week, with rest days interspersed between your training days. As this is the hardest program in the book, do not be disheartened if you cannot perform all of the movements at first. Progress will come, and with time you will notice your body getting stronger and more mobile.

17

Creating Your Own Programs

In this part of the book, we are going to look at designing your own programs. The ideas presented will help you to create a bespoke series of exercises to target your injuries or physical weaknesses. Injuries vary from person to person, so rehabilitation should focus on individual needs. All of us have niggles and injuries that are unique (to us) in terms of their locations, intensities and combinations. Note that this chapter has been written with the understanding that not everyone reading it will be highly experienced in either exercise or program writing. In other words, we want this chapter to be usable by even the most inexperienced reader.

First, it is essential that you know which area of your body you want (or need) to injury-proof. For example, if your primary physical activity or pastime is running and you find you are developing knee problems, you will most likely want to injury-proof the knees, in addition to the other lower body joints, such as the hips and ankles. There would of course be some benefit in performing the upper body movements, but since running impacts the joints of the lower body more, it would make sense that the exercises picked in this case are the lower body ones.

Second, your experience and ability will dictate which of the exercises you can include in your program. If we take the runner in the above example, they would be unwise to include the single-leg squat if they do not have the leg strength to perform it. If you are unsure of your ability level, simply start with the easiest movements and progress when you are ready. You will know it is time to move on when the exercises you are performing become too easy, or when the program no longer proves challenging.

Third, try to follow the recommended number of sets, number of repetitions or duration, and rest times listed in the programs, and adapt them if you need to. For example, if you find that three sets of push-ups are too much, drop to two sets and see how that suits. If you need 60 seconds of rest instead of 45 seconds, feel free to change this guide as well.

To finish, we have included, overleaf, a blank table for you to copy and use for designing your own programs. There is space to write the name of the program and the type of upper body, spine and lower body exercise, as well as the number of sets, the number of repetitions or the duration, and the amount of rest time between sets.

Program Name:			
	Sets	**Reps/duration**	**Rest**
Wrist exercises			
Elbow exercises			
Shoulder exercises			
Spine exercises			
Hip exercises			
Knee exercises			
Ankle exercises			

⓲
Frequently Asked Questions

In this chapter we answer some common questions that many people have concerning body-weight exercise and injury prevention/rehabilitation. If you have a specific query not addressed here, please email us at: bulletproofbodies@email.com.

Q1. I have never been injured. Why should I bother training to prevent injury?
A. You should think of training to prevent injury in the same way as taking out insurance on your house: you hope you do not need home insurance, but it is unwise not to purchase it. Training to prevent injury takes little time, but will do a number of things: apart from helping to prevent injury, it will build strength in areas of the body that traditional training might not develop, and it will allow improved physical function and performance in many areas of your daily life.

We have developed the exercises and training programs in this book to be performed as a warm-up to a more extensive workout, or as simple daily routines to carry out regardless of whether a more extensive workout is planned. This way, you will be insured against injury.

Q2. Is it OK for me to only do exercises for a specific joint or area?
A. This is fine, but we would also recommend overall conditioning for other areas of the body. Imbalances can and do occur, and these situations often require more training to correct. If you only have time to train a specific body part in your training session, include the relevant exercises from this book in that session, and aim to perform the exercises for the rest of the body parts on other relevant training days. Take, for example, a training strategy where you run on Monday, train arms on Wednesday and do core on Friday; you could then do injury prevention for the lower body on Monday, injury prevention for the upper body on Wednesday and spinal injury prevention on Friday. The exercises themselves do not take a huge amount of time, and can be easily built into a daily routine, once you know the exercises that give you most benefit.

Q3. I already have a warm-up routine. Can I simply replace my old routine with a program from this book?
A. Yes, this can be done, but only if the warm-up routine you are currently following does not help to prevent injury. If your current

warm-up is simply jogging on the treadmill for five minutes and then doing a few quick stretches, it is unlikely that your routine will target troublesome areas; it may even be contributing to your injuries. Always warm up the body prior to strength or flexibility work.

Q4. I am retired and not as mobile or strong as I used to be. Are the exercises in this book suitable for me?

A. The exercises in this book are suitable for every reader, regardless of age. We have graded the movements so that you know which ones are easier and which are more challenging. Furthermore, the order in which the exercises appear is also an indication of their difficulty. The exercises in this book are designed to help with loss of strength and mobility, and there is good evidence to suggest that these physical functions provide a greater quality of life in older age.

Q5. I already have a physiotherapist/physical therapist, and the exercises in this book differ from the ones they have given me. How do I know which exercises are going to work and which are not?

A. All registered physiotherapists/physical therapists will be qualified, and will have sufficient knowledge to assess injuries and rehabilitate them. They may not be familiar with body-weight exercise, either from personal experience or from their therapy training. This book therefore offers an alternative or adjunct to your standard physical therapy.

We approach injury prevention and rehabilitation from the perspective of making the body as strong, mobile and injury resistant as possible. The exercises in this book will encourage you to identify and work on any physical deficits you may be suffering from. If the program you are following does not have a global aim to maximise your physical function, it may be a good idea to supplement your current rehabilitation with the exercises in this book. We do not advocate discontinuing any prescribed exercise advice unless you feel it is the right thing to do.

Q6. I am pregnant. Are the exercises in this book safe for me?

A. The answer to this question is complicated: some of the exercises may be less safe than others. For example, some of the simpler stretches are obviously safer than the German hang, which requires you to support your own body weight from a bar while hanging upside down. In addition, some of the other exercises that require strong muscular contractions may raise blood pressure excessively. In preparation for childbirth, pregnancy can make ligaments much more lax than they would normally be, which could lead to injury with strenuous exercise. If you were to do any exercises from this book, we would advise only the low-level core stability exercises and stretches that do not position your body in such a way as to create unnecessary physical stress. If you are unsure, please ask your doctor or health professional whether it is safe for you to do any of these exercises. They will have knowledge of your unique situation and be able to advise accordingly.

Q7. I don't really have time to work out properly. Can I just do the injury prevention and rehabilitation routines from this book instead?

A. If you do not have enough time to train in a proper way, then yes, the routines and exercises in this book can be used on their own to maintain or improve your physical capabilities. Even though the actual injury prevention and rehabilitation exercises are great for building strength and mobility, the goal exercises for each chapter can be used very effectively as a proper workout routine on their own. For example, the shoulder chapter has the push-up, the triceps dip and the pull-up as goal exercises; these three movements are very good for building and maintaining a base of strength and fitness, and require very little time or equipment to perform. The same applies to all of the other muscle groups, and you can build a full routine out of the goal exercises.

Q8. I have had physical therapy/personal training before, and am comfortable using machines and other equipment for exercises. What makes body-weight exercise so special?

A. While machines and other similar equipment can be used fairly effectively, they take away a very important aspect of human movement – stabilisation and control. Movement in the real world takes place in three dimensions; this means that the joints are free to move in practically any direction, and it is down to the muscles and other connective structures to control this movement. With exercise machines, however, the movement is almost always two-dimensional; in other words, the machine guides the direction and limits the movement.

Imagine a chest press machine as an example. This machine consists of handles that can be pushed forwards against a resistance. There is only one path that the handles can take, and so the muscles and joints do not have to worry about controlling the weight, balance or anything that resembles a natural human movement. This exercise would develop chest strength that involves only pushing forwards, but this would not necessarily replicate any other movement in the real world.

If we compare the chest press to a push-up, it is immediately apparent that the push-up is a three-dimensional movement, since the shoulders are free to move forwards, backwards and sideways – in fact, any

direction they choose. Consequently, the push-up requires much more control than a pushing exercise on a machine. Moreover, consider the core strength needed to maintain the push-up position, and the control and stability required of the hips and legs. All this would give you an all-round workout in the same time that you could have worked only the chest on a press machine.

These facts are not hugely important if we are just talking about general training, but we are trying to prevent and rehabilitate injuries here. As this is the case, then three-dimensional exercises are exactly the kinds of movement that we should be carrying out, in order to strengthen and improve the control of the body as a whole. Body-weight exercise is especially good for this, because every movement that is performed by the body is three-dimensional. In addition, body-weight exercise can be scaled up and down and very easily.

Q9. I have a child who is injured. Are these exercises safe for them to perform?

A. This another complicated question: it depends on the child, their age and their current training background, and on the skill of the adult in supervising and guiding the child. In theory, many of the exercises would be suitable for teenagers to perform, but be aware that excessive or heavy exercise at a young age can lead to problems with the muscles and skeleton. Seek advice from a medical or health professional.

Q10. The exercises for the cervical spine are not that advanced. Are there more advanced cervical exercises out there, to develop a strong neck area?

A. It is true that the exercises for the cervical spine in this book are not very advanced. This is intentional for a very good reason: since we are not present when you are performing the movements, we cannot be certain that you are doing them correctly. This is not too much of an issue with the vast majority of the movements discussed; however, as the cervical spine area is very vulnerable and serious injury could result, we have decided to leave out many advanced cervical neck exercises. If you are interested in some advanced techniques, the best places to go are martial arts gymnasiums, and other gyms (or coaches) that specialise in contact sports; these will have both the equipment and the knowledge to be able to oversee your neck training in a safe environment. Many of the common neck problems actually require adjustments to posture in the chest and lower spinal regions, and so addressing these will avoid the need for intensive neck exercises.